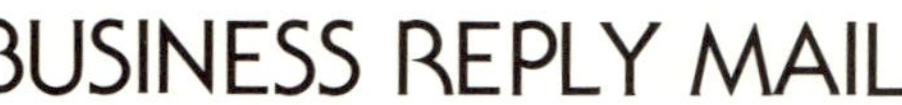

NO POSTAGE
NECESSARY
IF MAILED
IN THE
UNITED STATES

OTHER MONOGRAPHS IN THE SERIES, MAJOR PROBLEMS IN PATHOLOGY

Published

Evans and Cruickshank: *Epithelial Tumours of the Salivary Glands*

Mottet: *Histopathologic Spectrum of Regional Enteritis and Ulcerative Colitis*

Whitehead: *Mucosal Biopsy of the Gastrointestinal Tract*

Hughes: *Pathology of Muscle*

Thurlbeck: *Chronic Airflow Obstruction in Lung Disease*

Hughes: *Pathology of the Spinal Cord*

Striker, Quadracci and Cutler: *Use and Interpretation of Renal Biopsy*

Fox: *Pathology of the Placenta*

Asbury and Johnson: *Pathology of Peripheral Nerve*

Forthcoming

Azzopardi: *Problem Lesions of the Breast*

Frable: *Thin-Needle Aspiration Biopsy*

Hartsock: *Diagnostic Histopathology of Lymph Nodes*

Hendrickson and Kempson: *Surgical Pathology of the Uterine Corpus*

Lee and Ellis: *Bone Marrow Biopsy Pathology*

Lukeman and Mackay: *Tumors of the Lung*

Mackay: *Soft Tissue Tumors*

Panke and McLeod: *Pathology of Burn Injury*

Phillips: *Diagnostic Liver Pathology in Clinical Practice*

Sagebiel: *Histopathologic Diagnosis of Melanotic Lesions of Skin*

Smith: *Diagnostic Pathology of the Mouth and Jaws*

Warner: *Testicular Biopsy*

Whitehead: *Mucosal Biopsy of the Gastrointestinal Tract, 2nd ed.*

Woods: *Metabolic Diseases of Bone*

BASIL C. MORSON, M.A., D.M., B.M., B.Ch., M.R.C.P., F.C.Path.

Consultant Pathologist and Director of Research
The Pathology Department of St. Mark's Hospital
London

THE PATHOGENESIS OF COLORECTAL CANCER

Volume 10 in the Series

MAJOR PROBLEMS IN PATHOLOGY

JAMES L. BENNINGTON, M.D., *Consulting Editor*

Chairman, Department of Pathology
Children's Hospital of San Francisco
San Francisco, California

W. B. Saunders Company, Philadelphia, London, Toronto

W. B. Saunders Company: West Washington Square
Philadelphia, PA 19105

1 St. Anne's Road
Eastbourne, East Sussex BN21 3UN, England

1 Goldthorne Avenue
Toronto, Ontario M8Z 5T9, Canada

The Pathogenesis of Colorectal Cancer ISBN 0-7216-6558-6

 Made in the United States of America. Press of W. B. Saunders Company. Library of Congress catalog card number 78-1792.

Last digit is the print number: 9 8 7 6 5 4 3 2

CONTRIBUTORS

HENRY J. R. BUSSEY, B.Sc., Ph.D.

Consulting Research Fellow, St. Mark's Hospital, London.

J. W. COLE, M.D.

Director, Comprehensive Cancer Center and Division of Oncology, Yale University, New Haven, Connecticut

PELAYO CORREA, M.D.

Professor of Pathology, Louisiana State University Medical Center;

Attending Pathologist, Charity Hospital of New Orleans;

Consultant Pathologist, Veterans Administration Hospital, New Orleans, Louisiana.

DAVID W. DAY, M.A., M.B., B.Chir., M.R.C. Path.

Research Fellow, Department of Pathology, St. Mark's Hospital, London.

NORMAN MARTIN GIBBS, M.B., M.R.C.P., F.R.C. Path.

Hon. Professor of Pathology, University of Surrey;

Consultant Histopathologist, St. Luke's Hospital, Guildford, Surrey;

Hon. Research Fellow, St. Mark's Hospital, London.

MICHAEL J. HILL, Ph.D., M.R.C.Path. M.R.I.C.

Director, Bacterial Metabolism Research Laboratory, Central Public Health Laboratory, Colindale, London;

Consultant to the Research Department, St. Mark's Hospital, London.

D. KATZ, M.B.Ch.B., M.R.C. Path.

St. Mark's Hospital, London.

J. E. LENNARD-JONES, M.D., F.R.C.P.

St. Mark's Hospital, London.

BASIL C. MORSON, M.A., D.M., B.M., B.Ch., M.R.C.P., F.C. Path.

Consultant Pathologist and Director of Research, The Pathology Department of St. Mark's Hospital, London

ASHLEY B. PRICE, M.A., B.M., B.Chir. M.R.C.Path.

Consultant Histopathologist, Northwick Park Hospital and Clinical Research Centre, Harrow, Middlesex.

ROBERT H. RIDDELL, M.B., B.S., M.R.C.S.

Visiting Assistant Professor, Department of Pathology, The University of Chicago, Chicago, Illinois

JEAN K. RITCHIE, D.M., M.R.C.P.

St. Mark's Hospital, London.

D. C. SHOVE, M.B.Ch.B.(N.Z.), F.R.C.P.A.

Research Fellow in Histopathology, St. Mark's Hospital, London.

FOREWORD

"It has been our contention that the epithelial polyp-carcinoma relationship is not an inevitability. There are those who disagree with this view, feeling that there is a reasonably strong or strong relationship between epithelial polyps and carcinoma of the large intestine."[1]

"The observations that atypism, carcinoma-in-situ, or intramucosal carcinoma is rarely seen except in adenomatous polyps and papillary adenomas and that invasive foci less than 5 mm. in diameter are rarely seen except in these lesions, constitute evidence to support the belief that the vast majority of cancers arise in adenomatous polyps and papillary adenomas."[2]

During the last twenty years, there has been considerable controversy concerning the role of adenomatous polyps in the evolution of adenocarcinoma of the colon. The foregoing quotations give some indication of the divergent views on this subject which have been held by pathologists highly competent in morphology and research.

Dr. Basil Morson, a strong and longtime proponent of the adenoma-carcinoma sequence, and his co-authors speak with the authority of extensive research and vast experience on the subject of benign and malignant neoplasms of the colon and rectum. This book brings together in one source a complete and authoritative review of the clinical, morphologic, epidemiologic and experimental features of colonic polyps as well as the evidence this information provides in support of the concept that the adenomatous polyp is the precursor of colorectal carcinoma.

At a time when neoplasms of the colon represent a world-wide health problem of major proportion, pathologists, gastroenterologists, surgeons, epidemiologists and all others interested in this subject will find *The Pathogenesis of Colorectal Cancer* a timely and indispensable reference.

JAMES L. BENNINGTON, M.D.

1. Spjut, H.J. and Estrada, R.G.: The significance of epithelial polyps of the large bowel. (In) *Pathology Annual* 12, Part I, Appleton-Century-Crofts, New York, 1977, p. 166.
2. Grinnell, R.S. and Lane, N.: Benign and malignant adenomatous polyps and papillary adenomas of the colon and rectum. An analysis of 1,856 tumors in 1,335 patients. Surg. Gynec. Obstet. *106*:519, 1958.

PREFACE

Colorectal cancer is one of the more common forms of malignant disease, which is essentially curable if discovered in its early stages, and in theory preventable if detected in its precancerous phase. Research into its pathogenesis has revealed histopathological markers for patients at increased risk, markers which are valuable in clinical and epidemiological studies aimed at cancer prevention.

The main objective of this book is to describe the evidence in support of the concept that the colorectal adenoma is the most important precursor lesion for large bowel cancer. The approach to this is broadly based on clinical, histopathological, epidemiological and experimental evidence. Although the concept of the adenoma-carcinoma sequence has gained increasing acceptance in recent years, much of the evidence in its favour remains circumstantial and falls short of direct scientific proof. For this reason it is hoped that this book will be a stimulus to further research and a challenge to those who seek an alternative concept.

Basil C. Morson

ACKNOWLEDGMENTS

This book was conceived during the course of a conversation with Dr. James L. Bennington and I am most grateful to him and his team of reviewers for their help in finalizing the manuscript.

Gratitude is also due to all those clinical colleagues without whose co-operation the experience in this book could not have been so well documented. For many of the microphotographs I am indebted to Mr. Norman Mackie, senior photographer at St. Mark's Hospital, London, and Mr. W. Brachenbury, of the Department of Pathology, University of Nottingham. Miss D. Harwood gave much valued support in the typing of manuscripts and with proofreading. Finally, I would like to express my appreciation to the publishers and especially Mr. George Vilk for their efficiency and co-operation.

B.C.M.

CONTENTS

Chapter One

Introduction

Basil C. Morson

It is apparent that the incidence of cancer of the colon and rectum is increasing in the western World and among those populations who have adopted a western way of life (Segi and Kurihara, 1972; Berg and Howell, 1974). In the United States the incidence of the disease in the general population is greater than that of lung cancer and second only to skin cancer (Silverberg and Holleb, 1973). The surgical cure rate varies between 30 and 50 per cent in different centers and has changed little during recent decades. These facts make the study of the morphologic precursors, epidemiology, and etiology of large bowel cancer profoundly important because, short of accurate information about how any change in our environment might affect the incidence of this type of malignant disease, the clarification of precancerous states provides our best hope for cancer prevention.

At the present time there are three known predisposing causes of large bowel cancer: adenomas, familial polyposis, and ulcerative colitis. Polyposis and colitis contribute very little indeed to the total of patients who get cancer of the colorectum, but they are most useful models for cancer prevention. On the other hand, adenomas of the large bowel are very common. Their relationship to cancer is a most important issue that demands continued study in the hope that we will become better equipped to design cancer prevention programs.

Most of the confusion and disagreement over the classification and malignant potential of polyps of the large bowel results directly from controversies about nomenclature and the wrong use of words. For these reasons it is important to define accurately terms in current use and their synonyms.

It is essential in the first place to define the meaning of "polyp." This is a clinical term or gross description of any circumscribed tumor or elevation that projects above the surface of surrounding normal mucous

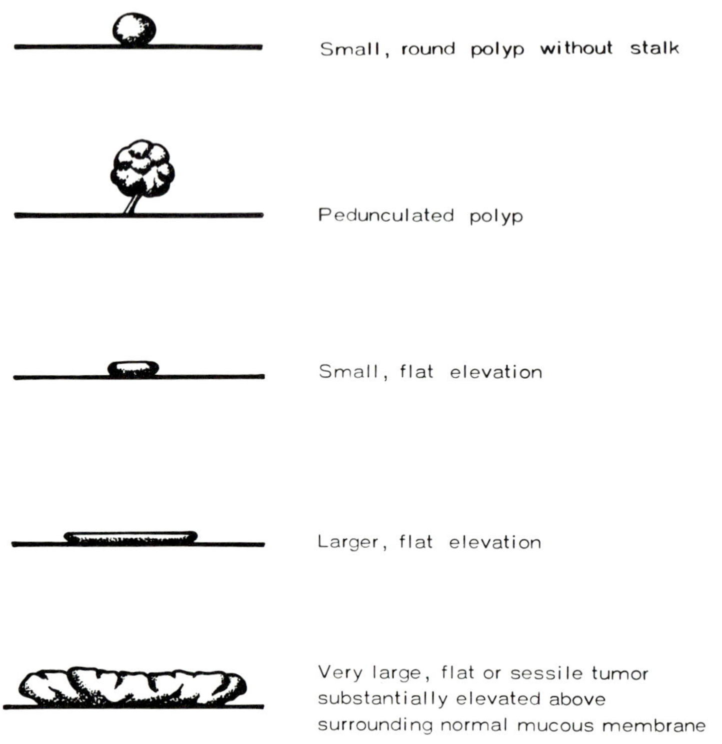

Figure 1–1.

membrane; it should *not* be used by itself as a histologic diagnosis. Figure 1–1 shows that polyps can be tumors on a long stalk, a short stalk, or no stalk at all. Less commonly they are flat or sessile elevations. Polyps with stalks are seldom larger than 3 cm in diameter, but sessile lesions can vary in size from a few millimeters in diameter to tumors as large as 10 cm across. The depth of elevation of sessile tumors above surrounding normal mucosa is also very variable. Although the shape and size of polyps are important to the surgeon and endoscopist from a purely technical point of view, histologic type has much greater significance.

There are many histologic types of polyp. These vary in their clinical significance and particularly in their malignant potential. It is essential that all removed polyps should be submitted to the histopathologist for microscopic examination because histologic type can have a very important bearing on the management of the patient. Fixation in formaldehyde solution must be prompt; any stalk should be identified with a thread tied around its base; and the larger sessile polyps should be pinned out flat on a small piece of cork board before being sent to the laboratory in fixative.

In Figure 1–2 a histologic classification is given of the common and most important benign polyps seen in clinical practice. There are others, of course, such as lipomas, which are not involved in the polyp-cancer controversy. There are four main classes, all of which can present as single or isolated multiple tumors or in the form of polyposis, a term usually reserved to describe the presence of hundreds or thousands of polyps covering the mucous membrane of the large bowel. Like "polyp" the word "polyposis" has significance only as a clinical or macroscopic term.

It is of the utmost importance to distinguish polyps of the large intestine with malignant potential from those that have no relationship to cancer. The adenoma group of tumors has malignant potential, and the evidence for this is given in subsequent chapters. Only the histopathologist can identify the different types, and the correct management of the individual patient with a polyp depends on accurate histologic diagnosis. In the following chapters the greatest emphasis is placed on the pathology of the adenoma-carcinoma sequence. Only an outline description is given of those types of polyp and polyposis that make no significant contribution to the relationship of polyps to cancer of the colorectum.

HAMARTOMAS

The hamartoma is a malformation composed of an abnormal mixture of tissues normally found in the affected part of the body—often with an excess of one particular tissue type. There is

HISTOLOGIC CLASSIFICATION OF POLYPS OF THE LARGE INTESTINE

Type	Single or Isolated Multiple Polyps	Polyposis
Neoplastic	Adenoma	Adenomatosis (familial polyposis)
Hamartomas	Juvenile polyp Peutz-Jeghers polyp	Juvenile polyposis Peutz-Jeghers syndrome
Inflammatory	Benign lymphoid polyp	Benign lymphoid polyposis Inflammatory polyposis e.g., in inflammatory bowel disease
Unclassified	Hyperplastic (metaplastic) polyp	Hyperplastic polyposis

Figure 1–2.

absolutely no evidence that isolated *juvenile polyps* or *Peutz-Jeghers polyps* have any malignant potential, although cancer has on rare occasions been reported in association with juvenile polyposis and the Peutz-Jeghers syndrome. At worst these two polyposis syndromes could be regarded as having a very low potential for cancer (see Chapter 8). The juvenile polyp has been called a juvenile "adenoma," but this is unfortunate because all the evidence suggests that it is not an "adenoma" in the sense of being a neoplasm. The old name "retention polyp" still is used occasionally, but is no longer in general favor. The evidence that the juvenile polyp is a hamartomatous rather than an inflammatory lesion is considered in both Chapters 3 and 8. The Peutz-Jeghers polyp has a characteristic histology for which fortunately no other nomenclature has been applied (see p. 27).

INFLAMMATORY POLYPS

The inflammatory group of polyps includes any that are clearly the consequence of an inflammatory disorder, such as ulcerative colitis, Crohn's disease, and dysenteric colitis. The expression "pseudopolyp" is used by some, but *inflammatory polyp* would seem to be a more logical term. There is nothing "pseudo" about any polyp, and inflammatory polyps are essentially the result of ulceration with undermining of adjacent mucous membrane and the formation of mucosal tags of varying shape and size.

The *benign lymphoid polyp* and *benign lymphoid polyposis* are included under this category because they are probably the consequence of an immunologic process itself promoted by infection and inflammation.

HYPERPLASTIC POLYP

(Synonym: Metaplastic Polyp)

Although the hyperplastic or metaplastic polyp has a distinctive histology, its nature remains obscure despite the interesting concept described in Chapter 2. For this reason it had best remain "unclassified" until its histogenesis is understood. In the United States the terminology "hyperplastic" is preferred, and this is quite acceptable provided that it is recognized that this polyp has no malignant potential and its histology is different from the adenoma group of tumors. At one time it was thought by some that this little tumor was related to cancer, and the term "metaplastic" was introduced to emphasize the banal quality of its histology.

THE ADENOMAS

The neoplastic group of polyps, better called adenomas or adenomatosis if they are multiple, can present to the radiologist, endoscopist, or histopathologist as isolated lesions or in the form of a polyposis. How many adenomas makes adenomatosis is a question that can be answered at present only by an arbitrary definition. Experience shows that patients with the rare disease known as "familial polyposis" or "polyposis coli" always have more than 100 adenomas in the large bowel, and usually hundreds or even thousands of these tumors (see Chapter 8). The number of patients with between 50 and 100 adenomas in the large intestine is very few indeed, but the range between 10 and 50 is more common. Multiple isolated adenomas between two and ten in number are, relatively speaking, a common occurrence.

The number of adenomas, whether presenting as solitary tumors or as multiple but isolated polyps, or in the form of a classic polyposis, is irrelevant to the problem of histologic classification. They are all adenomas and the expression "adenomatosis" may sometimes be preferred as an alternative term for familial polyposis.

There is a widespread belief that adenomatous polyps and villous adenomas are wholly separable tumors. In fact, these are only terms used to describe the extremes of a spectrum of histology in which there is an intermediate type, often called villoglandular or tubulovillous adenoma. In other words, they are different macroscopic and microscopic variants of one neoplastic process, and the word "adenoma" is applicable to them all. Although adenomas show these differences in tissue architecture it is important to emphasize that they have a common cytology. Indeed, this is the main reason for regarding the spectrum of histologic types only as different growth patterns of the one disease. The cytologic changes in adenomas are known as "epithelial atypia" or "dysplasia." Tubular adenomas, tubulovillous adenomas, and villous adenomas are separable by subjective microscopic criteria, but the more sections of any one tumor are examined, the more frequently the mixed or intermediate structure of tubulovillous adenoma is seen. The histology and cytology of adenomas are considered further in Chapter 5.

The World Health Organization (Morson et al., 1976) has recommended a preferred nomenclature based entirely on histologic structure (Fig. 1–3). Adenomas, whether single, few in number, or in many hundreds or thousands as in familial polyposis, are classified by their histologic structure into three groups. For adenomatous polyp the expression "tubular adenoma" is recommended because the tumor is composed of proliferating epithelial tubules. This terminology has the advantage both of accuracy and of omission of the contentious word "polyp." "Villous adenoma" is preferred to "villous papilloma" and "tubulovillous adenoma" for the villoglandular type, because it accurately describes those tumors that are intermediate in structure between

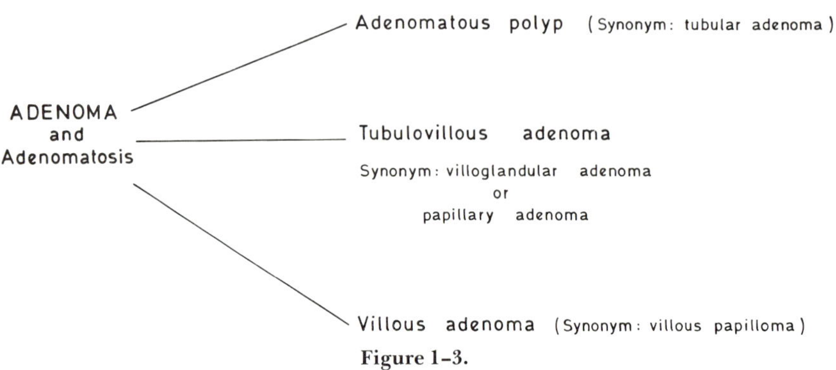

Figure 1–3.

tubular adenoma and villous adenoma. Whereas the latter has a villous growth pattern, some tumors have both tubular and villous components but usually very blunted villous processes. The term "papillary adenoma" has been used in the past as a synonym for the villoglandular adenoma as well as for villous adenomas.

It is essential to obtain agreement on the use of the word "carcinoma" or "cancer" in the context of malignant change in adenomas. By and large, "severe dysplasia" or "atypia" can be equated with the expression "carcinoma in situ." The meaning of this is readily understood among histopathologists but it can give a wrong impression when used in histologic reports. It communicates a sense of anxiety to some surgeons that can lead to unnecessarily radical operations. It cannot be emphasized too strongly that as long as tumor is confined above the line of the muscularis mucosae, there is no potential for metastasis even though the tissue changes satisfy all the cytologic criteria for adenocarcinoma. *Only when neoplastic epithelial cells have traversed the line of the muscularis mucosae is there any potential for metastasis.* The reason for this is that there are no lymphatics in colonic mucosa above the line of the muscularis mucosae (Fenoglio, Kaye, and Lane, 1973). For this reason it is best to restrict the use of the word "carcinoma" to that stage of the adenoma-carcinoma sequence which has crossed the line of the muscularis mucosae with invasion of the submucosal tissues. In these circumstances it is important to make the distinction from "pseudocarcinomatous invasion" (see page 54).

"Focal cancer" is an expression that should also be avoided because it is used by some to mean a focus of carcinoma in situ or severe dysplasia (atypia), whereas for others it means a focus of early invasion (microinvasion) across the muscularis mucosae into the stalk or submucosal tissues of a tumor that otherwise has the structure of an adenoma.

THE ADENOMA-CARCINOMA SEQUENCE AND CANCER PREVENTION

Provided certain important qualifications are borne in mind, there can be no doubt that adenomas, and villous adenomas in particular, have malignant potential and should be removed. At present many such tumors are found incidentally during examination for symptoms due to other conditions, or in operation specimens removed for cancer, diverticulitis, etc. It is the general clinical experience that these polyps are often symptomless, and this seems to be the most likely explanation for the fact that patients usually present with symptoms when malignant change has already taken place and, indeed, is often far advanced. After all, most patients with cancer of the colon and rectum have a history of symptoms for less than a year, and the evidence presented in Chapter 6 about the life history of the sequence would suggest that they have had the disease for at least five years prior to clinical diagnosis, and in many cases very much longer. The concept that cancer of the large bowel has a very long clinically latent phase before the patient presents for treatment is important, because it follows that cancer prevention can only be practiced effectively by identifying persons who are at increased risk from cancer but have no symptoms. How can such patients be identified? The identification of manageable populations of persons who are at increased risk from cancer of the large bowel is the only practical approach at the present time.

The adenoma marks a patient as being at increased risk from bowel cancer, but the size of this risk varies with the many different factors to be described in the following chapters. The objective should be to try to identify more accurately those groups of patients at the very highest risk, and concentrate scarce economic resources and technical expertise on them only. The adenoma is a very common tumor, and it is probably impracticable at present to register all adenoma-labeled individuals for purposes of follow-up and regular examination. On the other hand, prevention of colorectal cancer can be achieved in day-to-day clinical practice by identifying individuals who belong to known high-risk groups. For example, it is well known that patients who have had an adenoma or a cancer removed from one part of the colon or rectum commonly develop other such tumors in any remaining large intestine (see Chapter 7). It is for this reason that the discovery of an adenoma or a cancer anywhere in the colon or rectum should be followed by intensive investigation of the whole large bowel by barium enema or colonoscopy, or both. At present the air contrast enema would appear to be the cheapest and most effective technique, but colonoscopy obviously has an increasingly important role (Williams, Muto, and Rutter, 1973; Wolff and Shinya, 1974). Patients with adenomas or cancers have a significantly increased risk of producing further adenomas or cancers at some time during the rest of their lives. This means that all such patients (and this is a large, but probably still manageable population) should have regular follow-up examinations of any remaining large bowel at regular intervals. Study of the life history of the adenoma-carcinoma sequence suggests that this need not be more often than every three years provided the intestine was demonstrated as tumor-free at the previous examination. A group of patients at particularly high risk includes those who have had an operation for removal of multiple tumors, either benign or malignant, or both. It has also been shown that an adenomatous polyp or villous adenoma containing severe epithelial atypia is associated with an increased risk of associated cancer in another part of the large bowel (Kalus, 1972).

Even if the above policies were generally adopted there would still be a majority of patients with cancer of the colon and rectum seeking treatment for the first time at a relatively advanced stage of their disease. How can these persons be identified at an earlier stage of their disease? On the assumption, which is almost certainly correct, that most colorectal cancers and probably many adenomas bleed, an improved method has been introduced for the detection of occult blood in the stools (Greegor, 1972; Winawer, Sherlock, Schottenfeld, and Miller, 1976). The impregnated guaiac slide (Hemoccult) test answers many of the criticisms of the older methods of testing for occult blood. Further investigation will be needed to evaluate the application of this approach in the development of mass screening programs, but it could be argued that a positive Hemoccult test places a patient in a high-risk group for colorectal polyps or cancer, and this should be followed at least by sigmoidoscopy and barium enema, if not by colonoscopy. The numbers at risk in this way and therefore requiring further investigation might be very large, with a consequent strain on existing resources of money and expertise. Preliminary data, however, suggest that a screening test based on the potential for polyps and cancers to bleed has considerable promise in the detection of the adenoma-carcinoma sequence at a curable stage.

There is evidence that family studies can be helpful in the identification of patients at increased risk from bowel cancer. It has been shown, for example, that an early age of onset of the disease, the presence of adenomas as well as cancer in an operation specimen, and multiple synchronous cancers in patients, are all associated with an increased liability to cancer among the members of the patient's family (Lovett, 1974 and 1976). The practice of taking a detailed family history from all patients with colorectal adenomas and cancers should be encouraged; the discovery of a positive family history should be followed by identification, investigation, and indefinite follow-up of all other members at risk. "Cancer families" should be registered in the same way as "polyposis families" (Bussey, 1975), and members monitored at regular intervals at least by the Hemoccult test and sigmoidoscopy.

What is the relevance of the adenoma-carcinoma concept to the study of the cause or causes of large bowel cancer? If most cancers of the colon and rectum develop from pre-existing adenomatous polyps and villous adenomas, are the factors influencing the development of polyps the same as for cancers? Possible answers to these questions are given in Chapter 12. It would appear that many, if not most, adenomas never become malignant. Why some and not others? Here the example of familial polyposis is most vivid because, of the thousands of adenomas present, only one or a few cancers develop. Lastly, why is the life history of the adenoma-carcinoma sequence so variable? Many epidemiologic studies give strong support to the involvement of environmental factors in the etiology of cancer of the colon and rectum. By contrast, there are fewer studies of the epidemiology of precursor lesions (see Chapter 11). The evidence suggests that there is a statistical association between the prevalence of adenomas and the incidence of carcinoma of the colon. More such studies of the epidemiology of adenomatous polyps and villous adenomas are required in order to clarify the importance of the adenoma-carcinoma sequence on a geographic basis.

The evidence that variations in the composition of the bacterial flora of the intestine may be responsible for geographic variations in the frequency of large bowel cancer (Aries, Crowther, and Drasar, 1969; Hill, Drasar, and Aries, 1971; Drasar and Hill, 1972) has been reviewed in Chapters 11 and 12. Feces from persons in high-risk populations have higher counts of bacteroides and lower counts of aerobic bacteria than in populations in whom cancer of the colon and rectum is uncommon. Among the important metabolic activities of intestinal bacteria, particularly bacteroides, is the degradation of bile salts with the production of carcinogens, and it has been shown that the amount of substrate available for carcinogen production is greatest in the populations at high risk from bowel cancer. Application of this line of reasoning to small, manageable groups of patients with precursor lesions or with increased risk of bowel cancer could be fruitful. For example, those patients who have had one or more adenomatous polyps or villous adenomas removed from their bowel; patients with familial polyposis; those with total ulcerative colitis and a history of symptoms for more than ten years; and those who have had one cancer removed and, because of the presence of associated adenomatous polyps, are at particularly high risk from a second or metachronous bowel cancer. Does the composition of the bacterial flora influence the development of precancerous polyps as well as the onset of cancer?

Veale's hypothesis (Veale et al., 1966) provides a genetic basis for the etiology of isolated adenomas, multiple adenomas, and familial polyposis (see Chapters 8 and 12). This theory is not incompatible with the concept that important environmental factors are also at work in the production of the precursor lesions as well as the invasive cancer. The existence of "cancer families" in which the affected patients have few associated polyps, or none at all, is well-documented (Lynch and Krush, 1973). Such clustering of cancers has been explained on a genetic or an environmental basis, but it would seem more reasonable to suggest that for many patients both genetic and environmental influences are at work and that the way these interact determines the number of adenomas, their growth rate, and the liability to cancer (see Chapter 12).

CANCER PREVENTION IN POLYPOSIS

In the past it has become customary to regard polyposis as a wholly separate disease on the assumption that the adenomas present in this condition differed from those found as isolated lesions. Apparent differences have been reported (Leuchtenberger, Leuchtenberger, and Liebv, 1956; Birbeck and Dukes, 1963), but these have failed to stand up to closer scrutiny, and the only differences between the adenomas of polyposis and nonpolyposis patients would appear to be the number of tumors and possibly the mode of inheritance. This being so, it therefore would seem reasonable to regard polyposis with its heavy concentration of adenomas as a fruitful field for the study of the adenoma-carcinoma sequence.

In the investigation, treatment, and follow-up of polyposis families the important objective is to get affected individuals treated before they develop cancer. Cancer prevention has limited scope in the propositus group, as two-thirds of these patients already have cancer when first seen. The incidence of malignancy among the siblings, however, is less than that found in propositus family members and even more so among the children of affected members. The records of the St. Mark's Hospital Polyposis Register show a dramatic decrease in malignant disease among call-up family members as compared with the propositus group (see Chapter 8).

When polyposis is diagnosed before cancer has occurred, the adenoma-carcinoma sequence can be broken by surgical removal of the adenomas. This may be affected by either total proctocolectomy or colectomy and ileorectal anastomosis. The former makes certain that no further adenomas are produced, but leaves the patient with the permanent handicap of an ileostomy; the latter demands half-yearly review for the destruction of any polyps in the rectum. Moertel et al. report that this procedure carries a heavy risk of subsequent malignancy in the rectum, which they estimate to be an accumulative 59 per cent at 23 years after operation (Moertel, Hill, and Adson, 1970). This has not been confirmed by Schaupp and Volpe (1972), who record only one case of subsequent rectal carcinoma although 30 patients had been followed up for ten years or more. Bussey (1975) has also reported a lower figure of 3.6 per cent at 25 years, and although this has now risen to about 6.5 per cent, mainly owing to overenthusiastic conservation in a recent case, the risk can still be considered acceptable.

Since, in the absence of treatment, 50 per cent of polyposis patients can be expected to get cancer of the rectum, cancer prevention can be said to have been highly effective in the cooperative polyposis family up to the present, and should be even more so in the future. Indeed, with a complete record of all polyposis families and their total cooperation, it should be possible to reduce the incidence of associated cancer of the colon and rectum to a negligible figure. The good results obtained in the St. Mark's Hospital series not only provide evidence that the destruction of adenomas is an effective method of cancer prevention, but also point the way to a possible reduction of the incidence of intestinal cancer in the general population.

Although it seems certain that heredity plays an important role in the etiology of familial polyposis coli, it does not follow that cancer in these patients is also determined by heredity. It could be argued that the cancer develops because the patient is exposed to some environmental influence, although this would have to be of a ubiquitous nature since polyposis patients invariably develop one or more carcinomas if left untreated for long enough. Similarly, it cannot be presumed that the polyps in polyposis coli develop solely on a basis of heredity. The phenomenon of regression of adenomatous polyps in the rectum after colectomy and ileorectal anastomosis (Cole and Holden, 1959) suggests that environmental influences (changes in the bacterial flora, for example) could influence the growth of the polyps in these patients.

CANCER PREVENTION IN ULCERATIVE COLITIS

Most patients with colitis do not develop carcinoma of the large bowel. However, it is well-established that such tumors are more common in colitics than in the general population, and tend to occur at an earlier age. How great is the risk? Is it sufficiently great to advise a person with few or no symptoms to accept a major operation, often with the construction of a permanent abdominal stoma in order to prevent the onset of cancer?

Two trends may be discerned in the management of patients with extensive colitis (Lennard-Jones, Morson, Ritchie, Shove, and Williams, 1977). It is likely that carcinoma as a complication of colitis can be largely eliminated by advising proctocolectomy for all patients with extensive colitis, either early in the course of the disease for acute symptoms or after ten years in patients with mild disease (Bonnevie, Binder, and Anthonisen, 1974). This policy will increase the number of patients who undergo major surgery, most of whom will have to adjust to a permanent abdominal stoma. These operations have a mortality and morbidity both in the short (Watts, de Dombal, and Goligher, 1966a) and the long term (Watts, de Dombal, and Goligher, 1966b; Ritchie, 1971 and 1972), and excision of the rectum can lead to sexual dysfunction (May, 1966; Burnham, Lennard-Jones, and Brooke, 1977). The presence of a stoma can cause physical, psychologic, and social disability.

An alternative policy reserves operation for a patient with ill health due to colitis, or when the large intestine shows evidence of neoplastic potential as judged by histologic criteria (see Chapter 9). The evidence suggests that once consistent and severe epithelial dysplasia is recognized in a rectal biopsy carcinoma is often present, although the likelihood of surgical cure of early cancer is high. The success of this policy must depend on early recognition of dysplasia by frequent investigation, or perhaps by the development of new techniques, and on the fact that operation is advised at a stage when any cancer is curable.

Endoscopists may be able to develop techniques for recognizing areas of dysplastic or early neoplastic change so that directed biopsies or cytologic preparations can be obtained. The definition and grading of dysplasia requires further analysis, and observer variation needs assessment. Cytologic techniques (Levin, Riddell, and Kirsner, 1976) and the identification of carcinoembryonic antigen by immunofluorescence in biopsy specimens (Isaacson, 1976) merit further investigation.

References

Aries, V., et al.: Bacteria and the aetiology of cancer of the large bowel. Gut *10*:334, 1969.

Berg, J. W., and Howell, M. A.: The geographic pathology of bowel cancer. Cancer *34*:807, 1974.

Birbeck, M. S. C., and Dukes, C. E.: Electron microscopy of rectal neoplasm. Proc. R. Soc. Med. *56*:793, 1963.

Bonnevie, O., et al.: The prognosis of ulcerative colitis. Scand. J. Gastroenterol. *9*:81, 1974.

Burnham, W. R., Lennard-Jones, J. E., and Brooke, B. N.: Sexual problems among married ileostomists. Gut, *18*:673, 1977.

Bussey, H. J. R.: Familial Polyposis Coli. Johns Hopkins University Press, Baltimore, 1975.

Cole, J. W., and Holden, W. D.: Postcolectomy regression of adenomatous polyps of the rectum. Arch. Surg. *79*:385, 1959.

Drasar, B. S., and Hill, M. J.: Intestinal bacteria and cancer. Am. J. Clin. Nutr. *25*:1399, 1972.

Fenoglio, C. M., Kaye, G. I., and Lane, N.: Distribution of human colonic lymphatics in normal hyperplastic and adenomatous tissue. Its relationship to metastasis from small carcinomas in pedunculated adenomas. Gastroenterology *64*:51, 1973.

Greegor, D. H.: Detection of colorectal cancer using guaiac slides. Cancer *22*:360, 1972.

Hill, M. J., et al.: Bacteria and aetiology of cancer of the large bowel. Lancet *1*:95, 1971.

Isaacson, P.: Tissue demonstration of carcinoembryonic antigen (CEA) in ulcerative colitis. Gut *17*:561, 1976.

Kalus, M.: Carcinomas and adenomatous polyps of the colon and rectum in biopsy and organ tissue culture. Cancer *30*:972, 1972.
Lennard-Jones, J. E., Morson, B. C., Ritchie, J. K., Shove, D. C., and Williams, C. B.: Cancer in colitis: assessment of the individual risk by clinical and histological criteria. Gastroenterology, *73*:1280, 1977.
Leuchtenberger, C., Leuchtenberger, R., and Liebv, E.: Studies of cytoplasmic inclusions containing desoxyribose nucleic acid (DNA) in human rectal polypoid tumours including familial heredity type. Acta Genet. Statist. Med. *6*:291, 1956.
Levin, B., Riddell, R. H., and Kirsner, J. B.: Management of precancerous lesions of the gastrointestinal tract. Clin. Gastroenterol. *5*:827, 1976.
Lovett, E.: Familial factors in the aetiology of carcinoma of the large bowel. Proc. R. Soc. Med. *67*:751, 1974.
Lovett, E.: Family studies in cancer of the colon and rectum. Br. J. Surg. *63*:13, 1976.
Lynch, H. T., and Krush, A. J.: Differential diagnosis of the cancer family syndrome. Surgery *136*:221, 1973.
May, R. E.: Sexual dysfunction following rectal excision for ulcerative colitis. Br. J. Surg. *53*:29, 1966.
Moertel, C. G., Hill, J. R., and Adson, M. A.: Surgical management of multiple polyposis. Arch. Surg. *100*:521, 1970.
Morson, B. C., et al.: "Histological Typing of Intestinal Tumours," International Histological Classification of Tumours. No. 15. World Health Organization, Geneva, 1976.
Ritchie, J. K.: Ileostomy and excisional surgery for chronic inflammatory disease of the colon: a survey of one hospital region. Part I – Results and complications of surgery. Part II – The health of ileostomists. Gut *12*:528, 1971.
Ritchie, J. K.: Ulcerative colitis treated by ileostomy and excisioned surgery: fifteen years' experience at St. Mark's Hospital. Br. J. Surg. *59*:345, 1972.
Schaupp, W. C., and Volpe, P. A.: Management of diffuse colonic polyposis. Am. J. Surg. *124*:218, 1972.
Segi, M., and Kurihara, M.: Cancer mortality for selected sites in 24 countries. Japan Cancer Society, Tokyo, 1966–1967, No. 6., 1972.
Silverberg, E., and Holleb, A. I.: Cancer Statistics, 1973. Cancer *23*:2, 1973.
Veale, A. M. O., et al.: Juvenile polyposis coli. J. Med. Genet. *3*:5, 1966.
Watts, J. McK., de Dombal, F. T., and Goligher, J. C.: Early results of surgery for ulcerative colitis, Br. J. Surg. *53*:1005, 1966a.
Watts, J.McK., de Dombal, F. T., and Goligher, J. C.: Long-term complications and prognosis following major surgery for ulcerative colitis. Br. J. Surg. *53*:1014, 1966b.
Williams, C. B., Muto, T., and Rutter, K. R. P.: Removal of polyps with fibrooptic colonoscope: a new approach to colonic polypectomy. Br. Med. J. *1*:451, 1973.
Winawer, S. J., Sherlock, P., Schottenfeld, D., and Miller, D.: Screening for colon cancer. Gastroenterology *70*:783, 1976.
Wolff, W. I., and Shinya, H.: Modern endoscopy of the alimentary tract. Curr. Probl. Surg., Year Book Medical Publishers, Chicago, 1974.

Chapter Two

Hyperplastic Polyps

(Synonym: Metaplastic Polyp)

N. M. Gibbs, and D. Katz

Westhues in 1934 first recognized what he called the "hyperplastic polyp" as distinctive and separable from other varieties of colorectal tumor, and emphasized its essentially non-neoplastic nature. This small polyp is very commonly seen in the rectum by endoscopists, particularly in the neighborhood of carcinomas (Fig. 2–1), and this unfortunately led to the view that it was related to cancer. The very term "hyperplastic" had, for some, a neoplastic connotation. Morson (1962) introduced the term "metaplastic" polyp only to indicate a change from a normal to an abnormal epithelium, and because of the implications for excessive growth inherent in the word "hyperplastic." He also emphasized its essentially benign nature and lack of any relationship to either adenoma or carcinoma. This view has been supported by others (Wattenberg, 1959; Lane and Lev, 1963). Recent studies suggest that the epithelial cells of the hyperplastic polyp grow more slowly and live longer than normal mucosal cells, and can be regarded as "hypermature" (Hayashi et al., 1974).

CLINICAL FEATURES

Hyperplastic polyps are most common in the rectum, but are also found in all parts of the colon and occasionally in the appendix (Arthur, 1968; MacGillivray, 1972). They are nearly always multiple and can be present in such large numbers that they mimic the

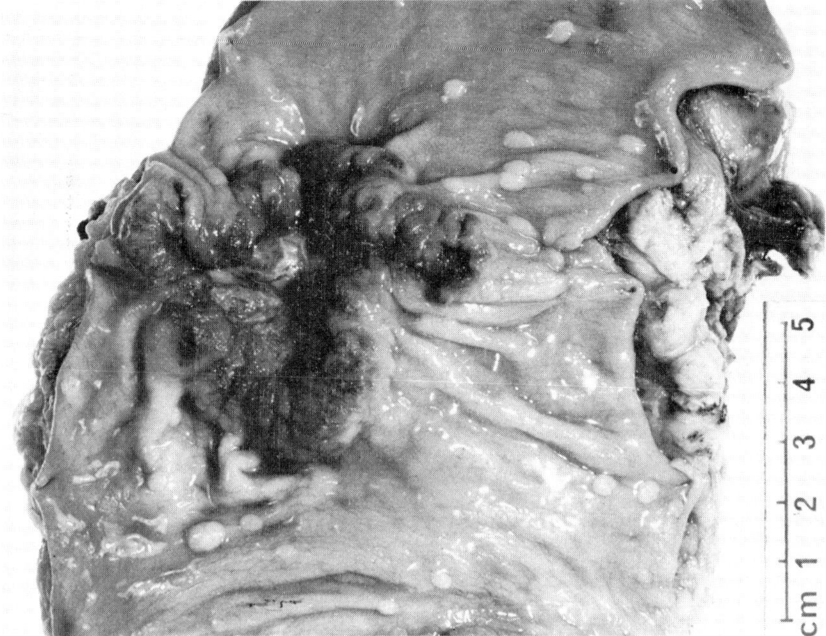

Figure 2–1 Hyperplastic polyps surrounding a carcinoma.

endoscopic and radiologic appearances of polyposis coli or adenomatous polyposis (see Chapter 8). Hyperplastic polyps are very common, increase in frequency with advancing years, and have been compared to senile hyperplasias in other sites, e.g., the skin. It has been estimated that they are present in about 40 per cent of adults of both sexes under 40 years of age and in 75 per cent over 40. They grow to a size of about 0.5 cm, very rarely larger. There is also clinical evidence that they can regress. The incidence of hyperplastic polyps is much greater in the rectum than in the remainder of the large intestine. One study of rectal hyperplastic polyps (Arthur, 1968) showed a high incidence in the middle third of the rectum, which coincides with the site where rectal carcinomas are most common. Analysis of the results, however, did not support any direct causal relationship between hyperplastic polyps and cancer.

The patient with a hyperplastic polyp often presents with symptoms referable to the large bowel, but these are usually due to an associated large bowel disorder, not to the polyp.

On sigmoidoscopy the size of hyperplastic polyps varies from 0.2 to 0.5 cm. The most common site is on the crest of the mucosal folds of either rectum or colon. They are usually sessile, the same color as or paler than surrounding normal mucosa, and with a flat or convex surface. Adjacent polyps may coalesce with each other or with adenomas and adenocarcinomas (Fig. 2–2).

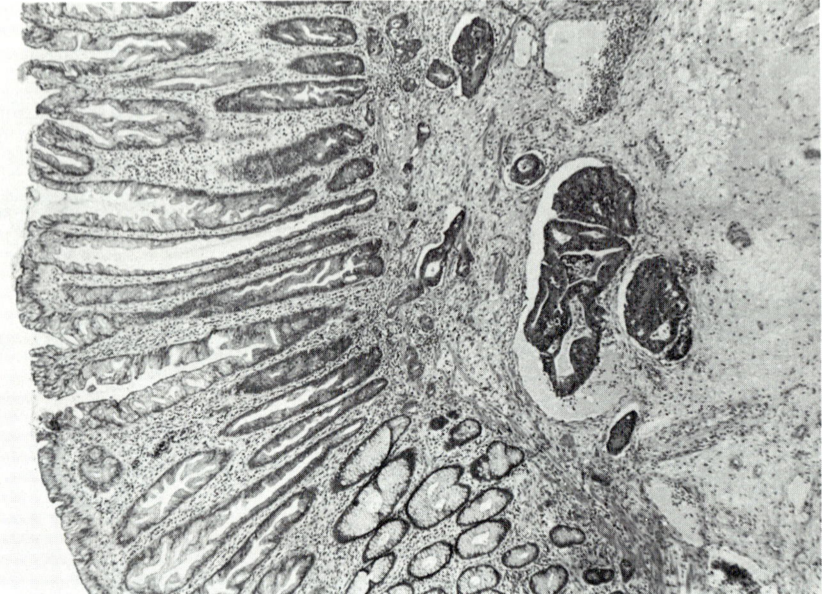

Figure 2–2 Hyperplastic polyp with submucosal lymphatic permeation from an adjacent adenocarcinoma. H & E × 40.

Histology

The hyperplastic polyp is clearly distinguishable from the adjacent normal mucosa (Fig. 2–3). The crypts are elongated and dilated. The goblet cells are normal but reduced in number. Absorptive cells predominate and these may show pseudostratification of nuclei (Fig. 2–4). Micropapillary processes (Fig. 2–5) protrude into the lumen of the crypts. The over-all appearance bears a marked resemblance to secretory endometrium (Fig. 2–6). The epithelial surface has a typical serrated appearance (Fig. 2–3). Argentaffin cells are prominent but situated in their normal position at the base of the crypts (Fig. 2–7). No Paneth cells are found. Mitoses are common but occur only at the base and in the lower midzone of the crypts. There is often a slight increase in lymphocytes and plasma cells in the lamina propria (Fig. 2–7). At the edge of the polyp the muscularis mucosae is often stretched and edematous, with dilated capillary channels.

PATHOGENESIS

Recent work by Kaye et al. (1973) and Hayashi et al. (1974), using the electron microscope and cell kinetic methods, has advanced our knowledge both of the normal behavior of the rectal epithelium and of the nature and significance of the hyperplastic polyp.

In normal rectal mucosa the epithelial cells originate at the base of the crypts. As they rise toward the surface, specialized characteristics develop, and at the surface there is exfoliation into the lumen; thus the most unspecialized cells are present at the crypt base. Already there are goblet cells in the lower third of the crypt with dense basal cytoplasm and a distended theca. The intermediate cells show extensive supranuclear apparatus and secretion droplets.

The middle third of the crypts is characterized by the maturation of absorptive cells with microvilli and basal-lateral intercellular convolutions. There are numerous mitochondria at the base of the cells. Toward the lumen the microvilli decrease in number, and the covering "fuzzy coat" with many "round structures" is lost. In these apical cells subcellular organelles are recognizable, such as transport vesicles, lysosomes, and microfibrils.

In vitro incubation of normal mucosa with tritiated thymidine reveals that the level of both the highest labeled cell in the individual crypt and the zone of maximal labeling density is in the middle third of the crypt by four to six hours. Over the subsequent 18 to 20 hours one can observe a steady rise toward the surface in both these parameters.

In the hyperplastic polyp the changes are quantitative rather than qualitative. At the base of the crypts there are already microvilli and intercellular apical desmosomes. These microvilli persist into the mid-

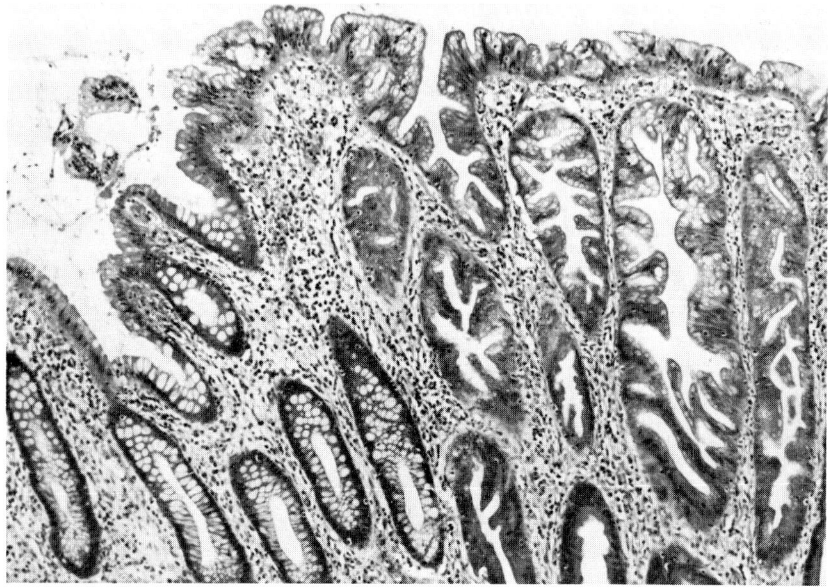

Figure 2–3 Hyperplastic polyp showing junction with normal colonic mucosa on the left. H & E × 63.

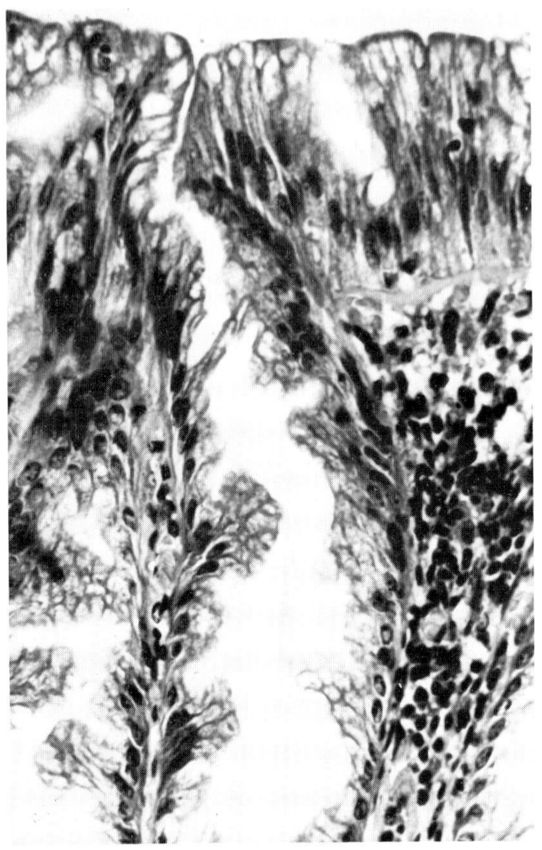

Figure 2–4 Serrated pseudostratified epithelium on the surface of a hyperplastic polyp. H & E × 200.

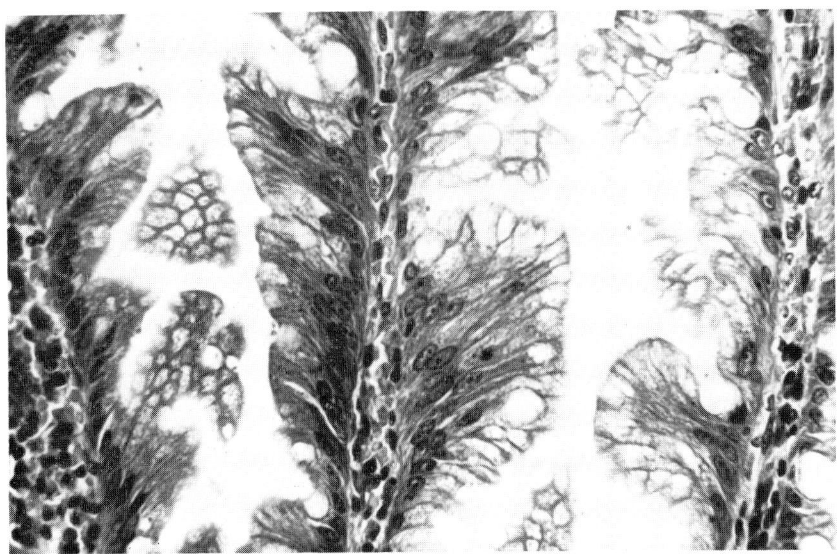

Figure 2–5 Micropapillae projecting into the lumen of a hyperplastic gland. H & E × 200.

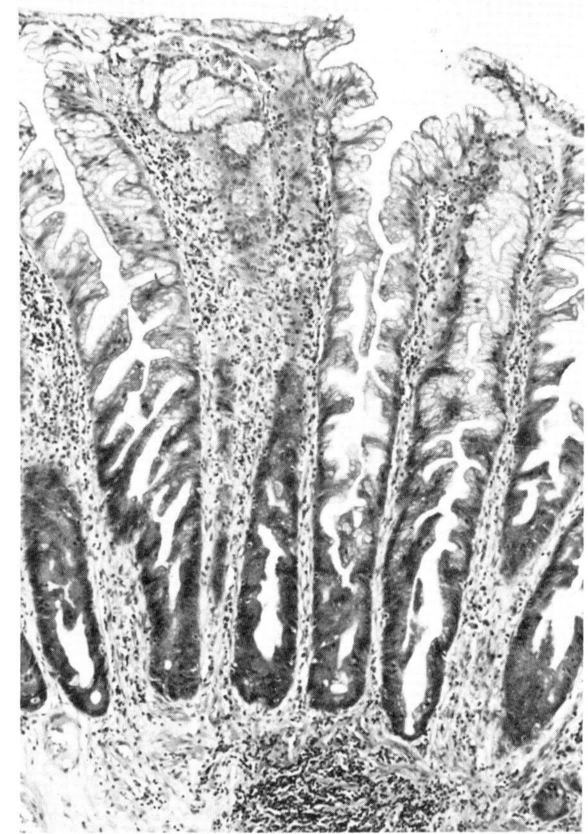

Figure 2–6 Dilated crypts of a hyperplastic polyp. H & E × 63.

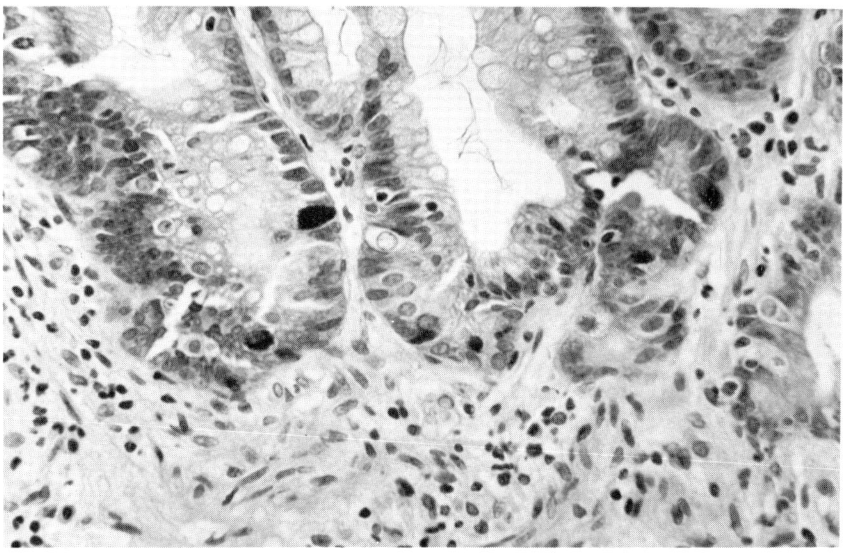

Figure 2–7 Base of crypt in a hyperplastic polyp showing normal argentaffin cells. H & E × 200.

portion, but are taller than normal with extended fibrillar cores protruding into the cytoplasm. The lateral convolutions are likewise exaggerated. At the surface of the crypts the cells have the membrane features of absorptive cells, but the intracellular features are those of aging with lipid and autophagic vacuoles. The widest separation of the cells by the lateral convolutions is found here. The normal blunting of microvilli and loss of the "fuzzy coat" does not occur.

The autoradiographic studies of hyperplastic polyps show that the migration of labeled cells is slower than normal; hence, the highest cell marked and the maximal uptake is nearer the base of the crypt at each corresponding time interval.

As these are changes in degree rather than character, it is not surprising that intermediate (or "early hyperplastic") appearances have been observed. These intermediate forms usually are not diagnosed macroscopically. Light microscopy shows "partial" disease with obvious changes apparent in only part of each individual crypt.

Similar studies on the adenomatous polyp show complete loss of orderly cell maturation. The cells are narrow and crowded, and show few poorly formed microvilli. Lateral convolutions are not present. DNA synthesis is random, with neither progressive rise from the base nor defined zone of maximal density.

In conclusion, the hyperplastic polyp, previously confused with adenomas and sometimes termed "metaplastic," can be defined as a separate entity representing an alteration in maturation of normal mucosal epithelium. The basal colonic epithelial cell acquires absorptive features lower in the crypt. DNA synthesis is less rapid. At the apex of the crypt cell maturation characteristics are accentuated. The factors that can produce this change in maturation are not known.

References

Arthur, J. F.: Structure and significance of metaplastic nodules in the rectal mucosa. J. Clin. Pathol. *21*:735, 1968.

Hayashi, T., Yatani, R., Apostol, J., and Stemmerman, G. N.: Pathogenesis of hyperplastic polyps of the colon: a hypothesis based on ultrastructure and in-vitro kinetics. Gastroenterology *66*:347, 1974.

Kaye, G. I., Fenoglio, C. M., Pascal, R. R., and Lane, N.: Comparative electron microscopic features of normal hyperplastic and adenomatous human colonic epithelium. Gastroenterology *64*:926, 1973.

Lane, N., and Lev, R.: Observations on the origin of adenomatous epithelium of the colon. Serial section studies of minute polyps in familial polyposis. Cancer *16*:751, 1963.

MacGillivray, J. B.: Mucosal metaplasia in the appendix. J. Clin. Pathol. *25*:809, 1972.

Morson, B. C.: Some peculiarities in the histology of intestinal polyps. Dis. Colon Rectum *5*:337, 1962.

Wattenberg, L. W.: A histochemical study of five oxidative enzymes in carcinoma of the large intestine in man. Am. J. Pathol. *35*:113, 1959.

Westhues, M.: Die pathologisch-anatomischen Grundlagen der Chirurgie des Rektumkarzinoms. Georg Thieme, Verlag, Leipzig, 1934.

Chapter Three

Juvenile and Peutz-Jeghers Polyps

N. M. Gibbs

JUVENILE POLYPS

Most juvenile polyps are found before the age of 20, although occasional cases have been described in old age (Mazier, Bowman, Sun, and Muldoon, 1974). Approximately three-quarters of juvenile polyps occur in the rectum, and most are situated within 5 cm of the anus (Toccalino, Guastavino, de Pinni, O'Donnell, and Williams, 1973). The remainder are found in the proximal large intestine, but they also occur occasionally in the stomach, small intestine, and appendix (Horrilleno, Ekert, and Ackerman, 1957). Juvenile polyps are usually single or few in number, but exceptionally large numbers are found in the stomach and intestine in the form of a gastrointestinal polyposis (see Chapter 8).

Symptoms characteristically develop in childhood during the first decade, with a peak incidence between 3 and 4 years. Many juvenile polyps are probably symptomless, and symptoms are related to the predilection of the polyp to undergo inflammation, ulceration, torsion, and autoamputation. Painless rectal bleeding immediately after defecation is the commonest symptom, and can be associated with the passage of the polyp in the stool. Polyps in the lower rectum may prolapse out of the anus. Multiple polyps are associated with iron deficiency anemia due to recurrent hemorrhage. Some inflammation is common in juvenile polyps, but there is no evidence that this is other than secondary to episodes of torsion of the pedicle and surface ulceration.

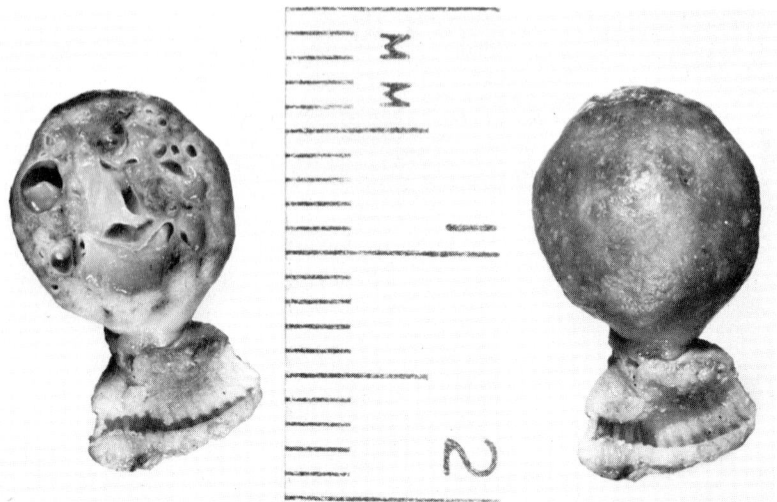

Figure 3–1 Macroscopic appearance of typical juvenile polyp showing smooth surface, short stalk, and cystic structure.

Macroscopic Appearance

Juvenile polyps are typically round in shape with a smooth surface, but a coarsely lobulated appearance tends to be adopted as a result of secondary inflammation and ulceration. In the fresh specimen, they have a bright red surface with patches of white due to the presence of underlying cysts filled with mucin (Figs. 3–1 and 3–2). The stalk is short and narrow. They vary in size from lesions of microscopic dimensions to tumors up to 2 cm in diameter. They are rarely any larger.

Microscopic Appearance

The surface of the typical juvenile polyp is covered by a single layer of columnar epithelium containing scattered goblet cells. This covering layer may appear cytologically normal, but is often modified by the effects of secondary inflammation so that it is usually attenuated or ulcerated. The substance of the polyp is formed by lamina propria, which is greatly increased in volume as compared with normal mucosa and the adenoma group of polyps (Fig. 3–4). The epithelial tubules, therefore, appear widely separated from one another and show tortuosity and cystic dilatation. They are filled with mucus and acute inflammatory cells (Fig. 3–3) which may rupture into the lamina propria (Fig. 3–5). The tubules are lined by tall columnar epithelium containing numerous goblet cells (Fig. 3–4). The tall epithelium is more prominent than adjacent normal colonic epithelium, and shows pseudostratification

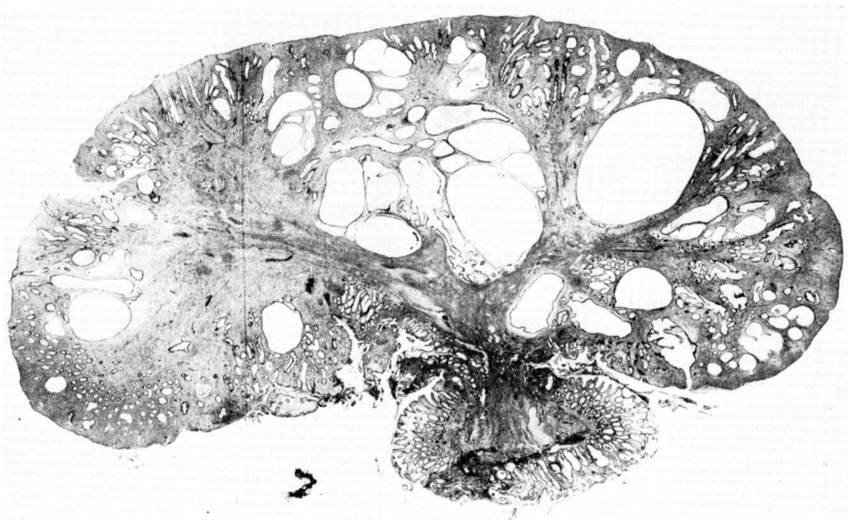

Figure 3–2 Low-power view of histology of juvenile polyp. The separation of cystic glands from one another by excess lamina propria is well shown. H&E × 6.4.

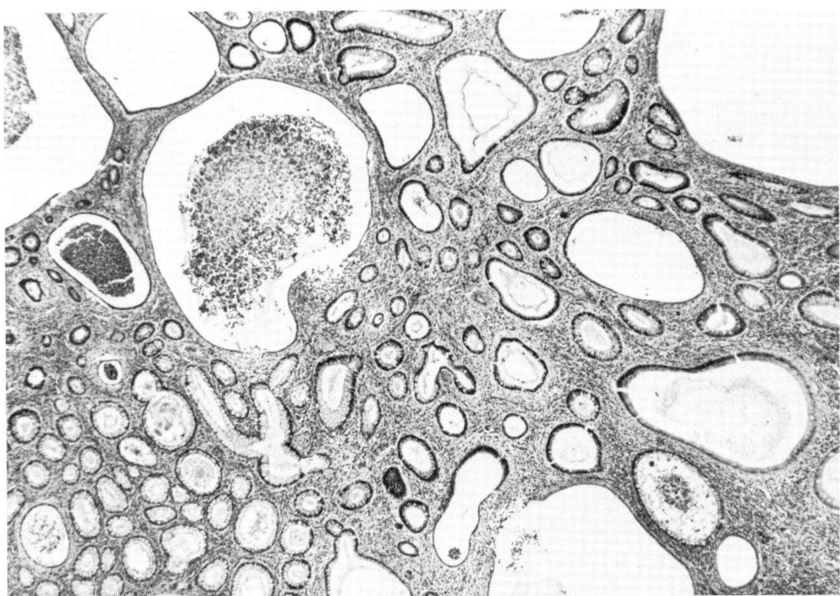

Figure 3–3 Histology of juvenile polyp. There is cystic dilatation of the glands, some of which contain mucin, inflammatory cells, and tissue debris. The glands are more widely separated from one another than in an adenoma, and are lined by non-neoplastic epithelium. H&E × 40.

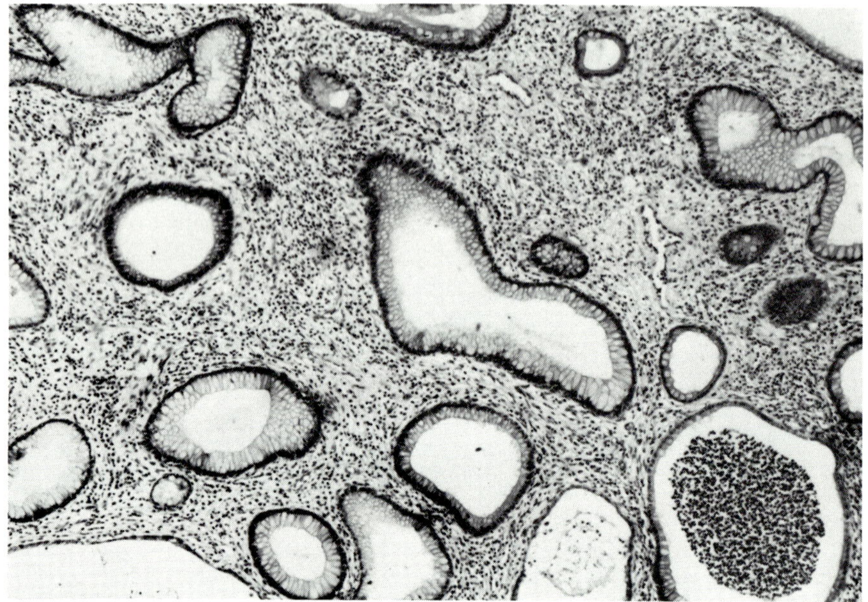

Figure 3–4 Histology of juvenile polyp showing cystic glands lined by somewhat normal-appearing epithelium, and separated by excess lamina propria. Some rather abnormal-appearing vascular channels can be seen in the lamina propria. H&E × 100.

of nuclei. Nevertheless, these are generally of normal size or slightly enlarged, and are aligned at the base of the cells. Mitoses are often increased in number. The cells populating the base of the glands (crypts) of the juvenile polyp appear normal (Fig. 3–5) and show a normal complement of argentaffin cells. Thus the epithelial changes are reactive to the secondary inflammation and are not neoplastic, but can be attributed to obstructive changes preventing drainage of mucus from the glands. The obstructed cystic glands are distended with mucin, inspissated secretion, necrotic cellular debris, and often acute inflammatory cells. Paneth cells are not seen in isolated juvenile polyps although they are common in juvenile polyposis (Gibbs, 1967).

The excess lamina propria has an edematous appearance (Fig. 3–4) and contains many dilated capillaries. The proteinous exudate in the interstitium may impart a diffuse pink tinge to sections stained with eosin. There is usually infiltration by an excess of inflammatory cells, although in the "pure" juvenile polyp without surface ulceration the number of inflammatory cells present in the excess lamina propria is no greater than normal.

It is not uncommon to see lymphoid follicles in the lamina propria of juvenile polyps, and bony metaplasia has also been described (Marks and Atkinson, 1964). Special stains do not reveal excessive collagen, but the extensive framework of reticulin demonstrates the excess of lamina propria. The muscularis mucosae does not participate in the histology of juvenile polyps as it does in hyperplastic polyps, adenomas, and especially polyps of the Peutz-Jeghers variety. The histology of the polyps in juvenile polyposis coli is described in Chapter 8.

It is important to recognize the histology of very small juvenile polyps. Pathologists rarely see them as solitary lesions because they probably do not give rise to symptoms, but they are readily studied in colectomy specimens removed for juvenile polyposis. The earliest histology (Fig. 3–6) appears to be a very few cystic tubules separated from one another by excess lamina propria and covered by a layer of columnar epithelium that, even at this early stage, may become attenuated and superficially ulcerated. Adjacent mucosa is normal.

Histogenesis

There are two theories. The first regards the polyp as a tumor produced by obstruction of the mucous glands through inflammation of the crypt orifices (Roth and Helwig, 1963). This concept of the inflammatory basis of juvenile polyps is based on histologic evidence alone.

The second theory is that the juvenile polyp is the result of a hamartomatous malformation affecting the glands and lamina propria,

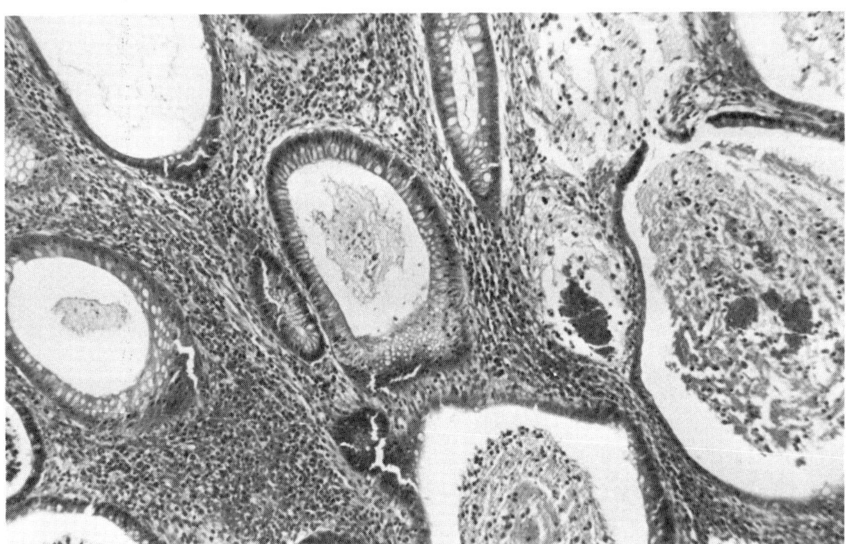

Figure 3–5 Histology of juvenile polyp. The tubules are cystic and one can be seen bursting into the lamina propria.

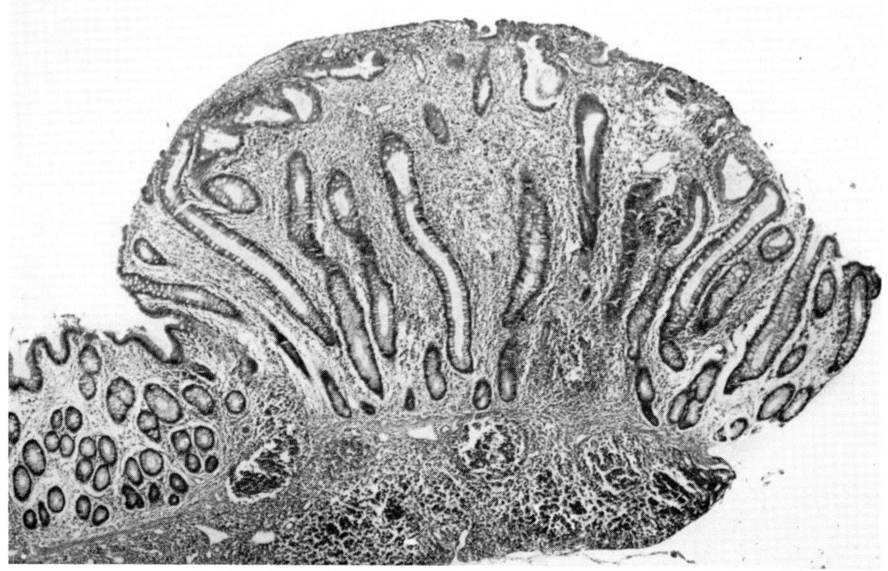

Figure 3–6 Histology of a very small juvenile polyp from a case of juvenile polyposis. The excess of lamina propria is apparent with lengthening and dilatation of the crypts. The lymphoid tissues beneath the muscularis mucosae are a coincidental finding. H&E × 30.

and that inflammation alone cannot be responsible (Morson, 1962). Support for the hamartomatous theory of origin comes from investigations using tissue culture techniques (Romer, Cotte, and Essenfeld-Yahr, 1971) and electron microscopy (Weller and McColl, 1966), both of which failed to demonstrate any abnormal epithelial elements or signs of neoplasm. It has been shown that juvenile polyps are composed essentially of normal tissues abnormally arranged, and that secondary ulceration, inflammation, and infarction can modify the histologic and cytologic features. The most prominent histologic feature in support of the hamartomatous theory of origin is a quantitative increase in the lamina propria as compared with the glandular component.

Furthermore, most juvenile polyps are found in infants and young children and are not associated with any inflammatory bowel disorder, and the mucosa adjacent to the juvenile polyps has a normal histology. The polyps of juvenile polyposis, however (see Chapter 8) are often associated with congenital abnormalities, and there is evidence of a genetic etiology. Veale (1965) has postulated that there is an allelic gene for the juvenile polyp, and that the genotype "P_j" accounts for the development of juvenile polyposis. Juvenile polyps have also been found in patients with other hamartomatous syndromes of the colon, such as polypoid ganglioneurofibromatosis (Donnelly, Sieber, and Yunis, 1969).

Malignant Potential

There is no evidence that isolated juvenile polyps ever undergo neoplastic transformation.

Differential Diagnosis

The juvenile polyp has a different macroscopic appearance from the adenoma. The surface of the juvenile polyp is smooth, unlike the adenoma which is crevassed. The lamina propria of the adenoma is not increased, but is encroached on by proliferating tubules. The normal crypt cells are displaced by the neoplastic cells of the adenoma, although normal argentaffin cells may be sequestrated. In contradistinction, cells of the crypts of the juvenile polyp appear normal. Hyperplastic and Peutz-Jeghers polyps have very different histologic appearances. Juvenile polyps must be distinguished from polyps occurring in inflammatory bowel disease, particularly ulcerative colitis. This distinction can be particularly difficult in juvenile polyposis; the reasons are not entirely clear, but are probably related to their susceptibility to ulceration and secondary inflammation.

HISTOLOGY OF PEUTZ-JEGHERS POLYPS

Peutz (1921) and Jeghers (1944) independently described cases of intestinal polyposis of a characteristic and uncommon type that is delineated in Chapter 8. It is not generally appreciated, however, that isolated polyps of the Peutz-Jeghers type are found in individuals who show none of the stigmata of the fully developed syndrome. These solitary polyps are as common as cases of multiple polyposis, and may be found anywhere in the stomach or intestine. In this chapter the pathology of Peutz-Jeghers polyps of the colon is described, regardless of whether they occur as solitary or multiple lesions.

Macroscopic Appearance

The polyps vary in size and can be large, reaching 3.5 cm or more in diameter. The larger ones are pedunculated and have a smooth, firm lobulated surface, not unlike some larger adenomatous polyps.

Microscopic Appearance

Peutz-Jeghers polyps are derived from intestinal glandular epithelium together with stroma that includes a muscular branching frame-

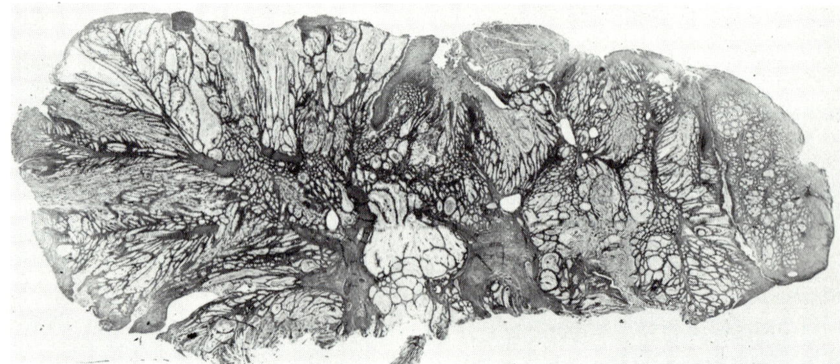

Figure 3–7 Peutz-Jeghers polyp of the colon showing branching bands of muscle derived from the muscularis mucosae and covered by mucus-secreting epithelium. H&E × 7.

work developed from the muscularis mucosae. Both the epithelial surface and the smooth muscle branching framework give the Peutz-Jeghers polyp the characteristic appearance (Figs. 3–7 and 3–8) that enables a diagnosis to be made by low-power microscopic examination of stained sections.

The glandular epithelium of the polyps resembles the parent mucosa (Figs. 3–7 and 3–8), and therefore colonic polyps are lined

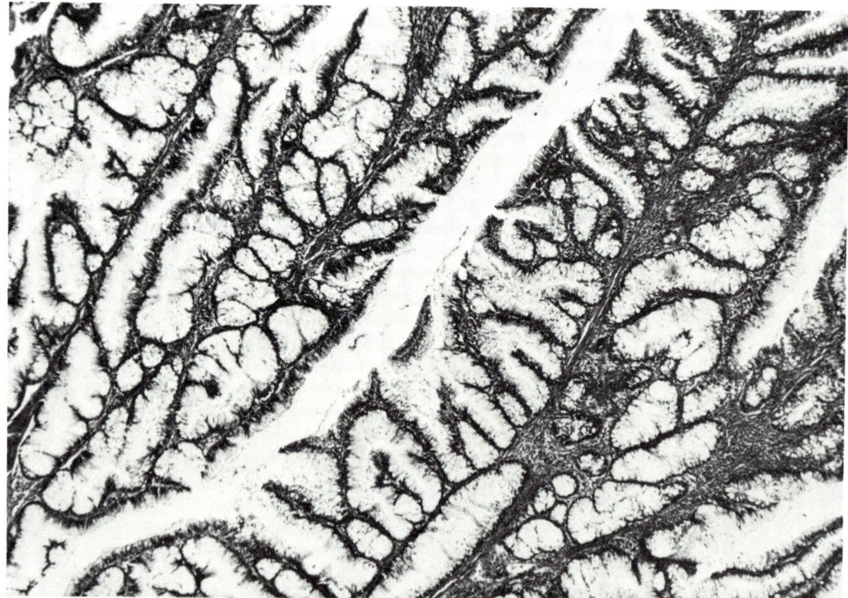

Figure 3–8 Peutz-Jeghers polyp of the colon. The branching bands of muscle are covered by mucin-secreting epithelium showing a minor degree of hyperplasia. H&E ×40.

predominantly by goblet cells. The crypts of each individual gland comprising the polyps are arranged close to the muscularis mucosae and appear cytologically normal, with a normal distribution of argentaffin (Fig. 3–10) and nonsecretory agranular cells (Gibbs, 1967). Some polyps can show scattered argentaffin cells throughout the glands. Paneth cells may also be present in the crypts, but they are not a prominent feature of colonic Peutz-Jeghers polyps.

The individual glands of the polyps are elongated and sometimes folded and convoluted (Fig. 3–8). The glands are composed of tall, mucus-secreting cells that have uniform nuclei situated basally (Fig. 3–9). The cells are sometimes crowded and can show some pseudostratification, and there may be a variation in cellularity between areas of the same polyp or between different polyps in the same patient. Likewise, mitotic activity is variable, but is only slightly increased by comparison with normal colonic mucosa.

Histogenesis

The presence of glandular overgrowth with a cytologic and structural resemblance to normal mucosa, together with the simultaneous development of an arboreal muscular framework derived from the muscularis mucosae, provides strong evidence for regarding Peutz-

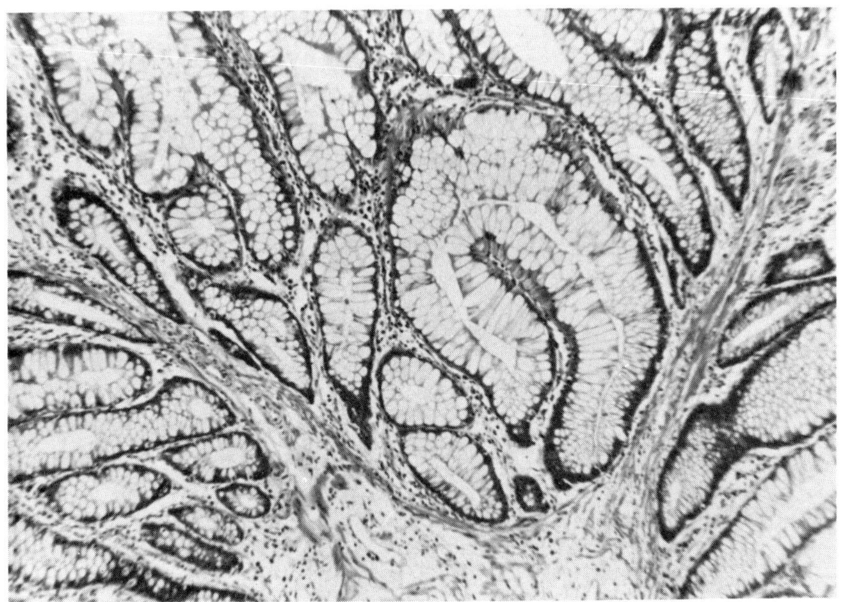

Figure 3–9 Base of Peutz-Jeghers polyp of colon showing the origin of the branching bands of muscle from the muscularis mucosae. H&E × 100.

Jeghers polyps as hamartomas (Bartholomew, Dahlin, and Waugh, 1957).

Malignancy

Peutz-Jeghers polyps are predominantly composed of epithelium, and as such represent a large population of cells growing in a restricted area. It can be postulated, therefore, on the basis of cell population per unit area of mucosa, that the chances of malignancy developing in a Peutz-Jeghers polyp are greater than in normal mucosa, on the assumption that the cells forming the polyps are equally liable as normal colonic cells to undergo neoplasia. However, in the colon there is good evidence to suppose that a large proportion of carcinomas develop from adenomas and are not derived from normal mucosal cells. Furthermore, adenomas may coexist with Peutz-Jeghers polyps in the same colon (Dodds, Schulte, Hensley, and Hogan, 1972), so that neoplastic transformation within a Peutz-Jeghers polyp must be demonstrated to provide conclusive proof. However, adenomas are rare in the stomach and small intestine, so that malignancy in Peutz-Jeghers polyps occurring in these sites is easier to substantiate.

It has been noted that the epithelium forming the glands of the Peutz-Jeghers polyp can appear hyperplastic and show increased mitotic

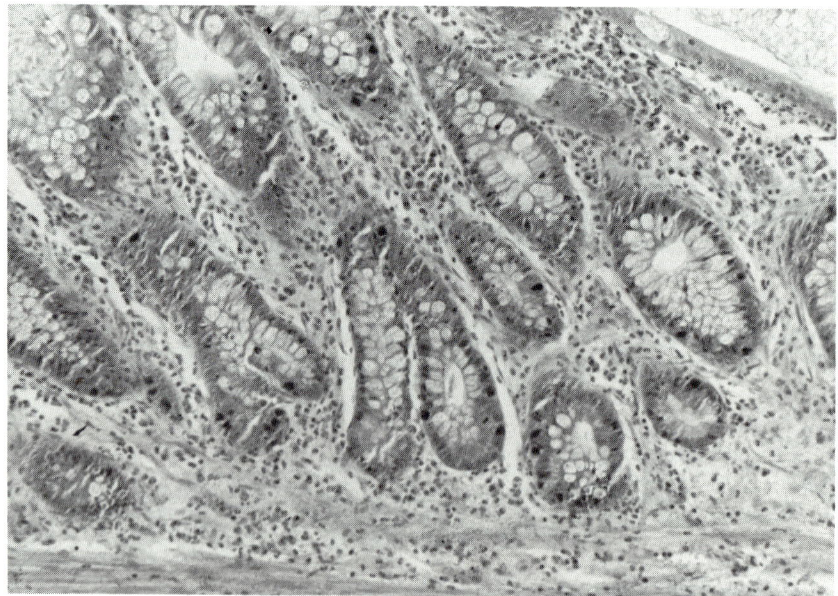

Figure 3–10 Numerous argentaffin cells in a Peutz-Jeghers polyp of the colon. Diazo reaction × 160.

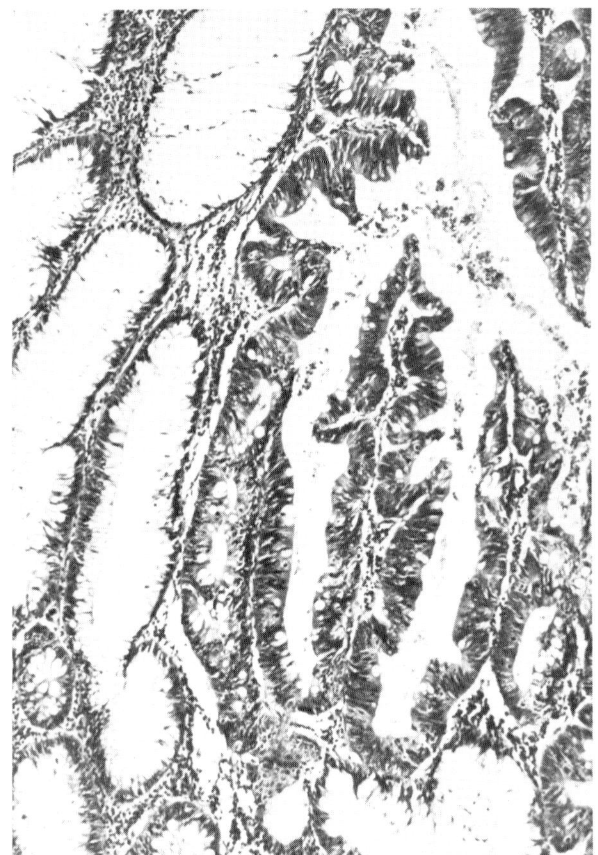

Figure 3–11 Epithelial dysplasia in a Peutz-Jeghers polyp of the colon. H&E ×60.

activity. However, the cellular abnormalities generally fall far short of the atypism present in adenomatous polyps. Occasional Peutz-Jeghers polyps show foci of dysplasia without invasion of the muscularis mucosae (Fig. 3–11), but this is excessively rare in the colon, and the author has only seen the one example illustrated here. Thus, it is conceivable that malignant change exceptionally could occur in Peutz-Jeghers polyps of the colon.

References

Bartholomew, L. G., Dahlin, D. C., and Waugh, J. M.: Intestinal polyposis associated with mucocutaneous melanin pigmentation (Peutz-Jeghers syndrome). Gastroenterology *32*:434, 1957.

Dodds, W. J., Schulte, W. J., Hensley, G. T., and Hogan, W. J.: Peutz-Jeghers syndrome and gastrointestinal malignancy. Am. J. Roentgenol. *115*:374, 1972.

Donnelly, W. H., Sieber, W. K., and Yuhis, E. J.: Polyps ganglioneurofibromatosis of the large bowel. Arch. Pathol. *87*:537, 1969.
Gibbs, N. M.: Incidence and significance of argentaffin and Paneth cells in some tumours of the large intestine. J. Clin. Pathol. *20*:826, 1967.
Horrilleno, E. G., Ekert, C., and Ackerman, L. A.: Polyps of the rectum and colon in children. Cancer *10*:1210, 1957.
Jeghers, N.: Pigmentation of skin. N. Engl. J. Med. *231*:88, 122, 181, 1944.
Marks, M. M., and Atkinson, K. G.: Heterotopic bone in a juvenile rectal polyp. Dis. Colon Rectum 7:345, 1964.
Mazier, W. P., Bowman, H. E., Sun, K. M., and Muldoon, J. P.: Juvenile polyps of the colon and rectum. Dis. Colon Rectum *17*:523, 1974.
Morson, B. C.: Some peculiarities in the histology of intestinal polyps. Dis. Colon Rectum *5*:337, 1962.
Peutz, J. L. A.: Very remarkable case of familial polyposis of mucous membrane of intestinal tract and nasopharynx accompanied by peculiar pigmentation of skin and mucous membrane. Nederl. Maandschr. V. Geneesk *10*:134, 1921.
Romer, H., Cotte, C., and Essenfeld-Yahr, R.: Behaviour of the rectal juvenile polyp in vitro. Gut *12*:194, 1971.
Roth, S. I., and Helwig, E. B.: Juvenile polyps of the colon and rectum. Cancer *16*:468, 1963.
Toccalino, H., Guastavino, E., de Pinni, F., O'Donnell, J. C., and Williams, M.: Juvenile polyps of the rectum and colon. Acta Paediatr. Scand. *62*:337, 1973.
Veale, A. M. O.: Intestinal Polyposis. Eugenics Laboratory Memoirs, Series 40, Cambridge University Press, London, 1965.
Weller, R. O., and McColl, I.: Electron microscopic appearances of juvenile and Peutz-Jeghers polyps. Gut 7:265, 1966.

Chapter Four

Benign Lymphoid Polyps and Inflammatory Polyps

A. B. Price

Although inflammatory polyps and lymphoid polyps are not involved in the pathogenesis of colorectal cancer, it is important for the histopathologist to recognize both of these entities and to be able to distinguish them from adenomas and malignant lymphomas.

INFLAMMATORY POLYPS

Ulcerative Colitis and Crohn's Disease

The most florid examples of this class of polyp occur in ulcerative colitis (Morson, 1968) and may be seen in 10 to 20 per cent of cases. They are seen less frequently in Crohn's disease (Schneider, Dickerson, and Patterson, 1973). The term 'pseudopolyp' is often used to refer to this particular complication, presumably to distinguish these lesions from the more sinister adenomatous polyps. However, the word 'pseudo' seems unnecessary; the lesions are polyps and the straightforward term "inflammatory polyp" is more accurate. They can be single or multiple, segmental or diffuse. Macroscopically they resemble wormlike outgrowths from the mucosa, with little distinction between stalk and head. They may have bifid ends or may form tubular bridges on the surface. The size varies from tiny nodules to arborescent structures 2 to 3 cm long (Fig. 4–1). In extreme cases the mucosal surface may resemble a mass of seaweed. In both Crohn's disease and ulcerative colitis the polyps predominate in the colon, rather than the rectum.

Histologically most are little more than mucosal tags consisting of a

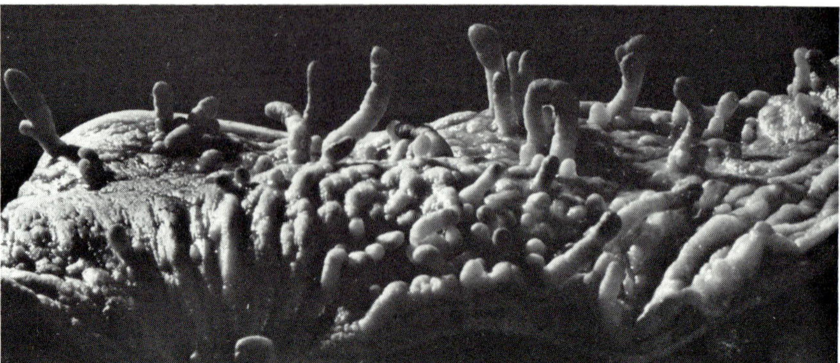

Figure 4–1 Inflammatory polyps in ulcerative colitis, the result of previous severe ulceration. There is no clear demarcation between the head and stalk, a helpful distinguishing feature from adenomatous polyps. (Photo: N. Mackie)

raised-up cylinder of mucosa along with muscularis mucosae and submucosa. The inflammatory infiltrate present is variable. In some cases the polyps are comprised of virtually normal epithelium (Fig. 4–2), but when inflammation is present the mucosal architecture is often disrupted. The glands can become cystic, show mucous depletion, and contain crypt abscesses. When this occurs, and especially if only a few

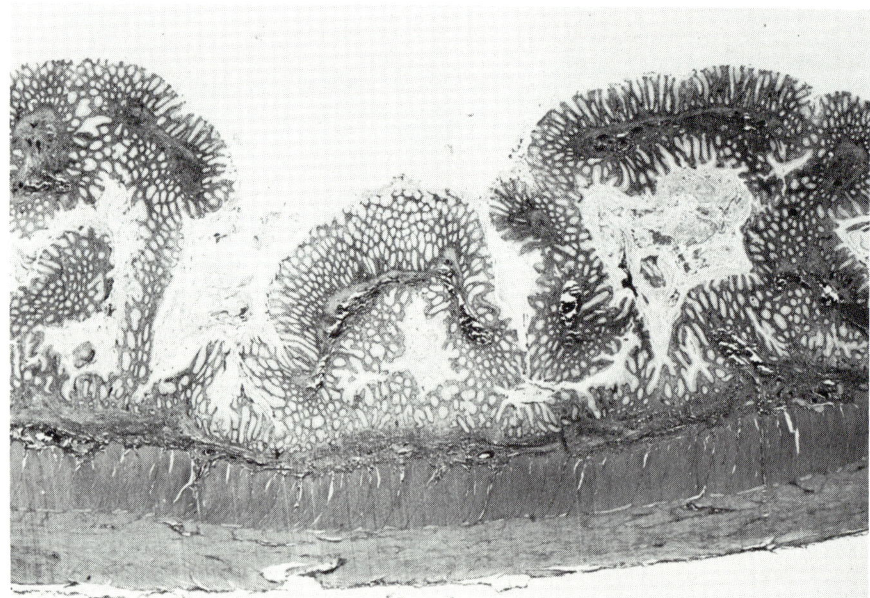

Figure 4–2 The mildly distorted mucosal architecture of the inflammatory polyp in ulcerative colitis. "Bridging" of the mucosa is seen, and in this case inflammation within the mucosal tags is minor. H & E × 11.

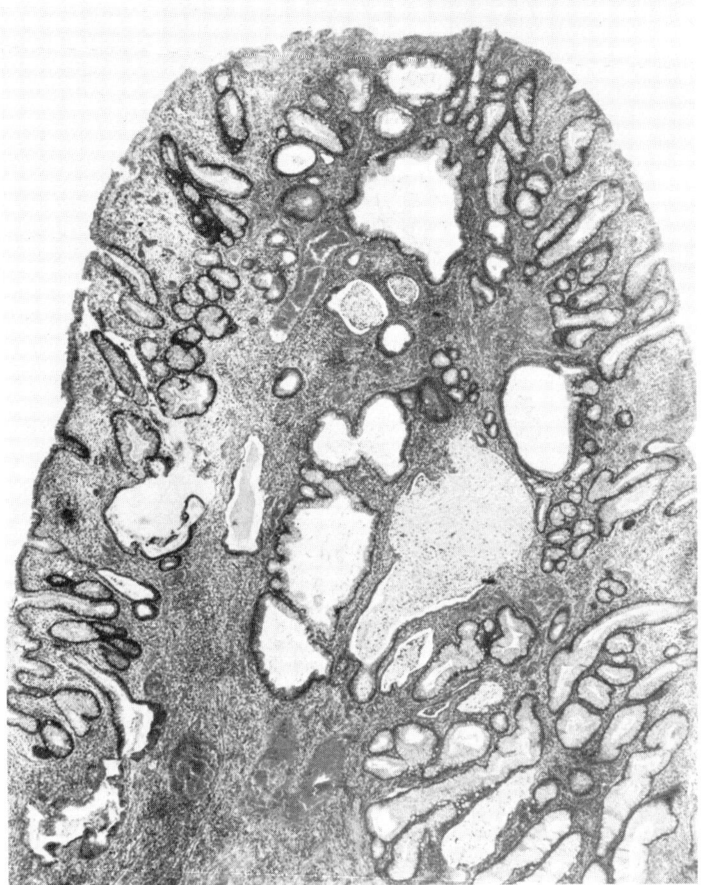

Figure 4–3 An inflammatory polyp with architectural distortion and more prominent inflammation than in Figure 4–2. Cystic glands are also present. This variety may be confused with the juvenile polyp, but here the background mucosal pattern is still evident. H & E × 30.

polyps are present, distinction from juvenile polyp can be difficult (Fig. 4–3). No muscularis mucosae is found in juvenile polyps, and mucus-filled cystic glands are conspicuous. The residual mucosal pattern is also less evident. Although it is generally believed to be a hamartomatous lesion, some workers still consider that the juvenile polyp has an inflammatory basis (Roth and Helwig, 1963). There should be little difficulty in distinguishing either of these forms of polyp from adenomas. Macroscopically these are usually sessile and carpet-like, or have a distinct stalk and lobulated head. On microscopy the glandular proliferation with varying degrees of dysplasia (fully described in Chapter 5 is also characteristic. The latter must not be confused with the glandular atypicality (reactive hyperplasia) sometimes seen in actively inflamed inflammatory polyps. The problem of distinguishing between true epithelial dysplasia (atypia) and reactive epithelial changes in the context of inflammatory bowel disease is dealt with in Chapter 9.

The occurrence of inflammatory polyps in nonspecific inflammatory bowel disease is related to at least one previous severe attack of colitis, in particular a total colitis. It is not related to the length of clinical history, but a positive association with toxic dilatation has been noted (Jalan, Walker, Sircus, and McManus, 1969). The suggested pathogenesis is that during a severe episode of colitis there is extensive full thickness mucosal ulceration with undermining of the surviving epithelium. Lengths of mucosa are stripped up and re-epithelialization occurs beneath, leaving these mucosal tags or "inflammatory polyps" projecting into the lumen. They may later rejoin the surface mucosa to form bridges, or arborize to form branched growths. The changes are believed to be irreversible.

Although early papers suggested such polyps in ulcerative colitis were precancerous (Dawson and Pryse-Davies, 1959), this is no longer accepted (Jalan, Walker, Sircus, and McManus, 1969) and they have no malignant potential. However, the polyps may mask a carcinoma on barium examination, or may mimic a carcinoma if solitary. In one series (Dawson and Pryse-Davies, 1969) 25 per cent of colitics with inflammatory polyps had solitary lesions. These cases pose a difficult problem for radiologists, and four of the six cases quoted were diagnosed as carcinoma. Clearly they can be confused with multiple adenomas or, in florid examples, familial polyposis. Colonoscopy and biopsy will settle the differential diagnosis. In particular the colonoscopist should biopsy any lesion with a distinct head and stalk. There are accounts of adenomatous foci arising within inflammatory polyps, and in one paper this incidence rose to 26 per cent (Goldgraber, 1965).

Inflammatory Polyps in Other Conditions

Beside Crohn's disease and ulcerative colitis, inflammatory polyps may occur in a wide variety of conditions, e.g., amebiasis (Berkowitz and Bernstein, 1975), schistosomiasis (Nebel et al., 1974), at anastomotic sites, near stercoral ulcers, etc. In these conditions the polyps are mostly rounded mucosal nodules. They have a granular surface unlike the lobulated pattern of adenomas, and seldom have a distinct stalk. Histology shows granulation tissue with a variable epithelial component (Fig. 4–4). Glands are scanty, and in infestations part of the parasite may be seen within the polyp. Unlike nonspecific inflammatory bowel disease, treatment of the particular condition results in regression of the polyps.

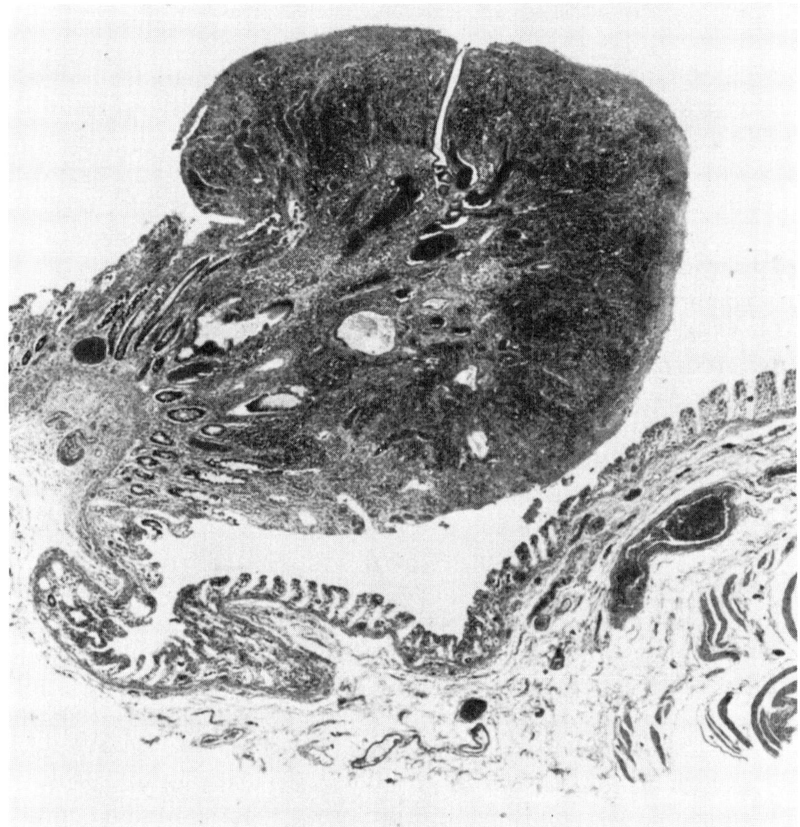

Figure 4–4 In this variety of inflammatory polyp the epithelial component is minor and the polyp is mainly granulation tissue. H & E × 18.

LYMPHOID POLYPS

Lymphoid tissue is present throughout the length of the gastrointestinal tract and plays a major role in the body's immunologic response. Particular concentrations are found in the hypopharynx, terminal ileum, and rectum where clusters of lymphoid follicles are present. The distinction between a physiologic and pathologic lymphoid response may be difficult, and an entire spectrum of change exists from isolated polypoid follicular lesions to diffuse lymphoid hyperplasia of the whole alimentary tract. The solitary benign lymphoid polyp of the rectum (Fig. 4–5), however, is the only form that pathologists will encounter regularly. It is also important to distinguish these benign lymphoid lesions from their malignant counterparts.

Benign Lymphoid Polyps

The benign lymphoid polyp (Hellwig and Hansen, 1951; Cornes, Wallace, and Morson, 1961) occurs most frequently in the lower one-third of the rectum in the third and fourth decades of life. Although it is usually solitary, several may be found, but more than six is rare. Many are discovered incidentally at rectal examination, but bleeding, constipation, and pain are common symptoms. The average size is 0.5 to 1.0 cm in diameter, but exceptionally they may grow as large as 3 cm. Approximately 25 per cent are stalked, the remainder being sessile mucosal nodules. Whether they are discovered incidentally or not, a biopsy is necessary. This must be of adequate size to enable the pathologist to distinguish a benign, and consequently unimportant, lesion from a malignant lymphoma. Should the lesion be benign, polypectomy may be performed if symptoms dictate. However, many will regress if left untreated. Such cases can be considered the extranodal counterpart of reactive follicular hyperplasia.

ETIOLOGY

The etiology of these solitary benign lesions is not clear, nor indeed whether they are truly pathologic, rather than exaggerated physiologic, responses (Hayes and Burr, 1952). No convincing evidence exists to suggest that they are neoplastic; inflammation of lymphoid tissue in other sites, and the occurrence of a comparable follicular proctitis in some cases of ulcerative colitis (Fig. 4–6), makes an inflammatory etiology the most acceptable (Holtz and Schmidt, 1958; Cornes, Wallace, and Morson, 1961).

Multiple Benign Lymphoid Polyposis

Multiple benign lymphoid polyposis of the large bowel is a recognized, if rare, entity (Shaw and Hennigar, 1974). Undoubtedly some recorded cases that regress spontaneously represent an exaggerated nonspecific physiologic change in the lymphoid tissue of the gut. It is usually a condition of young children, in contrast to the single lesions, and in keeping with the frequent hyperplasia of lymphoid tissue found in the young (Louw, 1968). Macroscopically the mucosa bulges with multiple gray sessile nodules from 0.3 to 0.6 cm in diameter. The importance of the condition lies in the differential diagnosis. Like the benign solitary lesion, it must be clearly distinguished from diffuse malignant lymphomatous polyposis of the intestine and also from familial (adenomatous) polyposis. If not, unnecessary colectomy may be carried out (Collins, Falk, and Guibowe, 1966; Gruenbarg and Mackman, 1972). With the advent of double contrast barium enemas

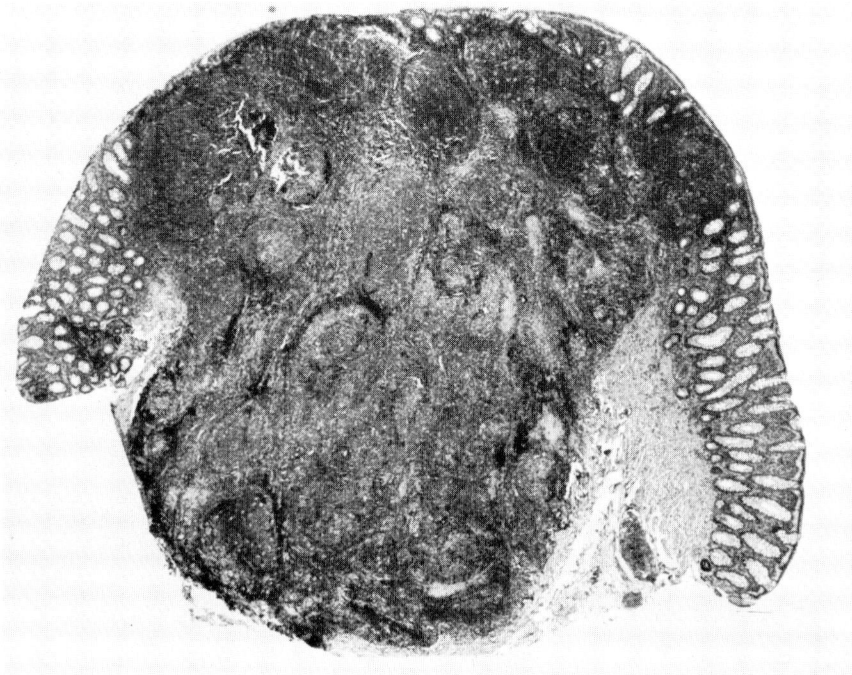

Figure 4–5 A benign lymphoid polyp. Note the well-circumscribed follicles with germinal centers that extend into, but not beyond, the submucosa. H & E × 18.

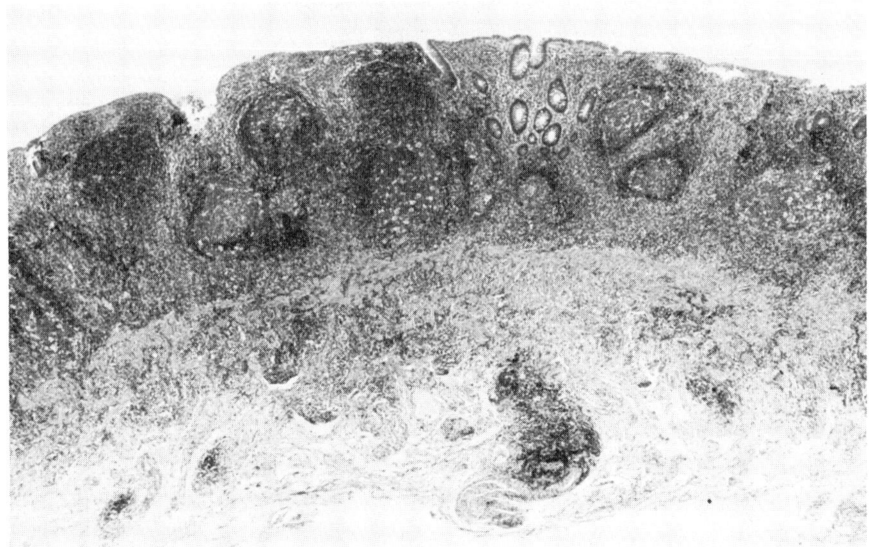

Figure 4–6 Follicular proctitis in a case of chronic ulcerative colitis. Note the discrete follicles with clearly demarcated germinal centers and the limited depth of the changes. H & E × 60.

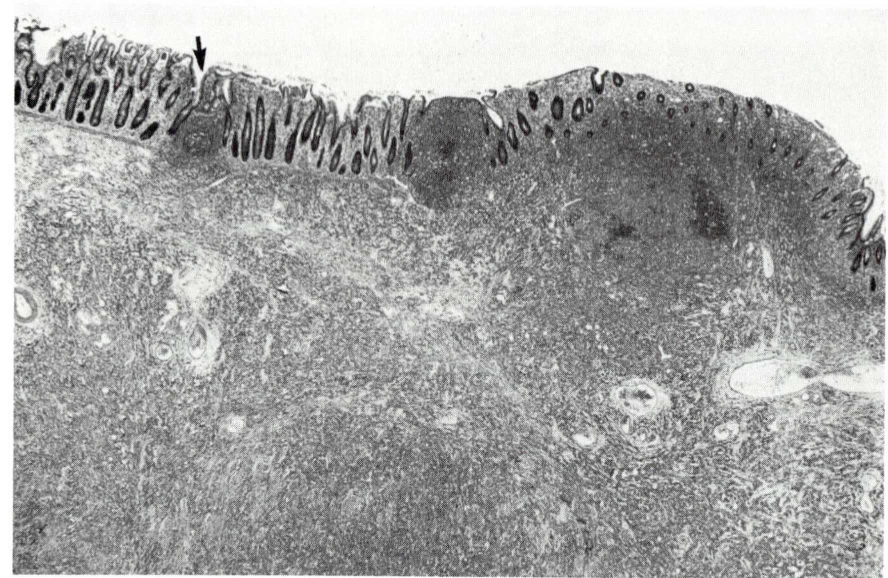

Figure 4–7 Malignant lymphoma of the colon. There is a diffuse lymphocytic infiltrate in the mucosa and submucosa that extends down into the muscle. One surviving nonmalignant lymphoid follicle with a germinal center is arrowed. H & E × 22.

and colonoscopy, minor degrees of diffuse lymphoid hyperplasia giving a polypoid appearance to segments of the mucosa are now accepted as normal, especially in the rectum in children (Franken, 1970; Robinson, Padron, and Rywlin, 1973). When symptoms occur, of which spontaneous hemorrhage is the commonest, multiple biopsies are essential.

A familial form of benign lymphoid polyposis has been described (Louw, 1968), and there is an increased association with familial polyposis. The terminal ileum is a frequent site of lymphoid polyposis in this class of patient (Bussey, 1975). Nodular lymphoid hyperplasia of the gastrointestinal tract is also seen in patients with immune deficiency syndromes (Shaw and Hennigar, 1974; Hermans et al., 1966).

The Histologic Differentiation Between Benign and Malignant Lymphoid Lesions

The criteria for distinguishing benign from malignant lymphoid lesions (Hellwig and Hansen, 1951; Dawson, Cornes, and Morson, 1961) in the intestine are similar to those employed for lymph nodes. The benign lymphoid polyp exhibits a follicular pattern with clearly defined germinal centers (Fig. 4–5). Usually at least three follicles are present; the pattern is regular and accompanied by adjacent broad bands of collagen. The lesion is centered on the submucosa, with mitoses and phagocytosis visible at the centers of the follicles. Foci of other inflammatory cells may be seen. As the polyp enlarges the overlying mucosa becomes attenuated, but rarely ulcerated. One of the radiologic signs of a benign lesion is a central dimpled area due to this flattening of the mucosa (Capitanio and Kirkpatrick, 1970). Extension in the muscularis propria is a rare feature of benign lymphoid lesions in the rectum, and when it occurs extra caution is required in assessing the other features. However, Saltzstein (1969) points out that this is seen in benign gastric lymphoid polyps, and is not therefore a malignant sign per se. Malignant lymphomas show only a poorly defined and irregular follicular pattern, with no germinal centers and no phagocytosis (Fig. 4–7). Except for cases of Hodgkin's disease, there is a monomorphic cellular infiltrate, other inflammatory cell types being rare. The lesions are poorly delineated with peripheral spread along the mucosa and through the muscle coat. Surface ulceration and fissuring are common. The resultant inflammatory response can partially obscure the lymphomatous infiltrate. In all cases, however, adequate tissue must be provided so that the above criteria may be assessed.

References

Berkowitz, D., and Bernstein, L. H.: Colonic pseudopolyps in association with amoebic colitis. Gastroenterology *68*:786, 1975.

Bussey, H. J. R.: Familial Polyposis Coli. Johns Hopkins University Press, Baltimore, 1975.

Capitanio, M. A., and Kirkpatrick, J. A.: Lymphoid hyperplasia of the colon in children. Radiology *94*:323, 1970.

Collins, J. O., Falk, M., and Guibowe, R.: Benign lymphoid polyposis of the colon. Pediatrics *38*:897, 1966.

Cornes, J. S., Wallace, M. H., and Morson, B. C.: Benign lymphomas of the rectum and anal canal. J. Pathol. Bacteriol. *82*:371, 1961.

Dawson, I. M. P., Cornes, J. S., and Morson, B. C.: Primary malignant lymphoid tumours of the intestinal tract. Br. J. Surg. *49*:80, 1961.

Dawson, I. M. P., and Pryse-Davies, J.: The development of carcinoma of the large intestine in ulcerative colitis. Br. J. Surg. *47*:113, 1959.

Franken, E. A.: Lymphoid hyperplasia of the colon. Radiology *94*:329, 1970.

Goldgraber, M. A.: Pseudopolyps in ulcerative colitis. Dis. Colon Rectum *8*:355, 1965.

Gruenberg, J., and Mackman, S.: Multiple lymphoid polyps in familial polyposis. Ann. Surg. *175*:552, 1972.

Hayes, H., and Burr, H. B.: Benign lymphomas of the rectum. Am. J. Surg. *84*:545, 1952.

Hellwig, E. B., and Hansen, J.: Lymphoid polyps (benign lymphoma) and malignant lymphoma of the rectum and anus. Surg. Gynecol. Obstet. *92*:233, 1951.

Hermans, P. E., et al.: Dysgammaglobulinemia associated with nodular lymphoid hyperplasia of the small intestine. Am. J. Med. *40*:78, 1966.

Holtz, F., and Schmidt, L. A.: Lymphoid polyps (benign lymphoma) of the rectum and anus. Surg. Gynecol. Obstet. *106*:639, 1958.

Jalan, K. N., Walker, R. J., Sircus, W., and McManus, J. P. A.: Pseudopolyposis in ulcerative colitis. Lancet *2*:555, 1969.

Louw, J. H.: Polypoid lesions of the large bowel in children with particular reference to benign lymphoid polyposis. J. Pediatr. Surg. *3*:195, 1968.

Morson, B. C.: *In* Goligher, J. C., de Dombal, F. J., Watts, J. McK., and Watkinson, G. (eds.): Ulcerative Colitis. Baillier, Tindell and Cassell, London, 1968, Chap. 2.

Nebel, O. T., et al.: Schistosomal disease of the colon: a reversible form of polyposis. Gastroenterology *67*:939, 1974.

Robinson, M. J., Padron, S., and Rywlin, A.: Enterocolitis lymphofollicularis. Arch. Pathol. *96*:311, 1973.

Roth, S. I., and Helwig, E. B.: Juvenile polyps of the colon and rectum. Cancer *16*:468, 1963.

Saltzstein, S. L.: Extra-nodal Malignant Lymphomas and Pseudolymphomas. *In* Sommers, S. C. (ed.): Pathology Annual No. 4. Appleton-Century-Crofts, New York, 1969, p. 159.

Schneider, R. S., Dickerson, G. R., and Patterson, J. F.: Localized giant pseudopolyposis. A complication of granulomatous colitis. Am. J. Dig. Dis. *184*:265, 1973.

Shaw, E. B., and Hennigar, G. R.: Intestinal lymphoid polyposis. Am. J. Clin. Pathol. *61*:417, 1974.

Teague, R. H., and Read, A. E.: Polyposis in ulcerative colitis. Gut *16*:792, 1975.

Chapter Five

Pathology of Adenomas

David W. Day and B. C. Morson

PREVALENCE, DISTRIBUTION, AGE, AND SEX

Adenomas, with the exception of hyperplastic (metaplastic) polyps, are the commonest type of polyp found in the colon and rectum. However, their prevalence in the general population is not accurately known. The marked variation in published series is explained first by the varying selection bias used in different studies, and second by the nature and adequacy of the studies themselves. Thus, factors such as the age distribution of the population examined, and whether symptoms related to the gastrointestinal tract are present, obviously affect prevalence figures. Even in asymptomatic people such as those who attend cancer detection clinics, for example, selection probably plays a part; those with a family history of cancer are more likely to attend than those without. Socioeconomic factors also may influence the composition of such a group.

Examination of the whole of the colon and rectum, and a histologic study of any polyps found, is essential to determine the prevalence of adenomas. Hyperplastic polyps, before their recognition as a separate entity, were included in the adenoma group. Series based on surgical material overemphasize rectal and sigmoid lesions because of cases diagnosed during routine proctosigmoidoscopic examinations; those based on roentgenologic appearances alone are unreliable in that small polyps are undetectable by this method of examination, and the designation of a polyp as an adenoma requires histologic confirmation.

Autopsy studies provide the most accurate information on the prevalence of adenomas, although again some selection bias is inevitably present, and the rapid autolysis of the gastrointestinal tract after death can interfere with accurate histologic diagnosis. As pointed out by Chapman (1963), an important reason for the wide discrepancy in the published figures from various autopsy series (from 7 to 51 per cent) is the fact that the autopsies were performed by a number of prosectors, and the results obtained retrospectively. Reliance can be placed only on series in which the examinations have been carried out by one person. It is also a laborious task to examine minutely the whole of the large intestine and to section every mucosal abnormality, and some authors have restricted histologic study to polyps over a certain size. Other factors to be borne in mind when comparing the results of different studies are the possible influence of time-trends and geographic variations on the prevalence of adenomas (see Chapter 10).

Chapman (1963), in his study of 443 consecutive autopsies on individuals over the age of 10, found adenomatous polyps in 226 cases or 51 per cent. In 99 cases there was one polyp only, and in the remainder there were two or more. The likelihood of an adenoma being present rose with increasing age, so that in the 60 to 80 age-group 50 to 60 per cent had one or more adenomas. In the series as a whole the distribution of these tumors in the large intestine was as follows: cecum, 7 per cent; ascending colon, 33.9 per cent; transverse colon, 28.4 per cent; descending colon, 8.8 per cent; sigmoid colon, 18 per cent; rectum, 3.9 per cent. This distribution, however, altered from age 50 to 60, in which the sigmoid colon was the most common site, to age 60 to 80, in which the ascending colon became the site of greatest prevalence. It is not clear from Chapman's paper, however, whether hyperplastic polyps were included.

In another autopsy study (Blatt, 1961) adenomas were found in 38.8 per cent of 446 colons from persons over 30 years of age, the numbers increasing with the age of the subjects, and over one-half of the total occurring in the 70 to 89 age-group. In 58 per cent of cases more than one adenoma was present, and in 35 per cent more than two. The distribution was: cecum, 18 per cent; ascending colon, 19 per cent; transverse colon (including the hepatic and splenic flexures), 25 per cent; descending colon, 11 per cent; sigmoid flexure (that part of the left colon subtended by a mesentery), 20 per cent; rectum, 7 per cent. Fifty per cent of the adenomas were 0.5 cm or less in diameter, and 84 per cent were 1.0 cm or less in diameter. Only 2.3 per cent had a diameter greater than 2.0 cm. Of the 75 polyps larger than 1.0 cm in diameter, 20 were present in the cecum and 24 in the sigmoid flexure.

Arminski and McLean (1964) calculated from the data in their autopsy series that 23.7 per cent of the male adult population and 24.2 per cent of the female adult population would have adenomas. They found two-fifths of the adenomas in the right and left halves of the colon respectively, and one-fifth in the rectum. Approximately 60 per cent of all adenomas were less than 0.5 cm in diameter, 25 per cent were between 0.5 and 1.0 cm, and 15 per cent were over 1 cm, these figures agreeing closely with those of Blatt. They found that the ratio of large to small polyps was greater in the left colon than the right. The authors estimated that 8 per cent of adults have polyps over 0.5 cm in diameter and 4 per cent have adenomas over 1 cm in diameter.

One point that emerges from all these autopsy studies is that adenomas are uncommon before the age of 30 but thereafter are present with increasing frequency as a population ages. Another is that the distribution of adenomas throughout the colon is much more even than clinical series had suggested. Most series report a slight but definite male predominance.

There is a need for further observations on the prevalence of adenomas, with particular reference to their histologic growth patterns and size at the various anatomic sites of the colon.

MACROSCOPIC AND MICROSCOPIC

Adenomas of the colon have a variable macroscopic appearance, and when a large number are studied all gradations are seen, from the tubular adenoma at one end of the spectrum to the villous adenoma at the other. The typical tubular adenoma (Fig. 5–1) is small, spherical, and pedunculated, with a smooth surface broken into lobules by intercommunicating clefts. The villous adenoma, on the other hand, is usually large and sessile with a shaggy surface made up of numerous fronds

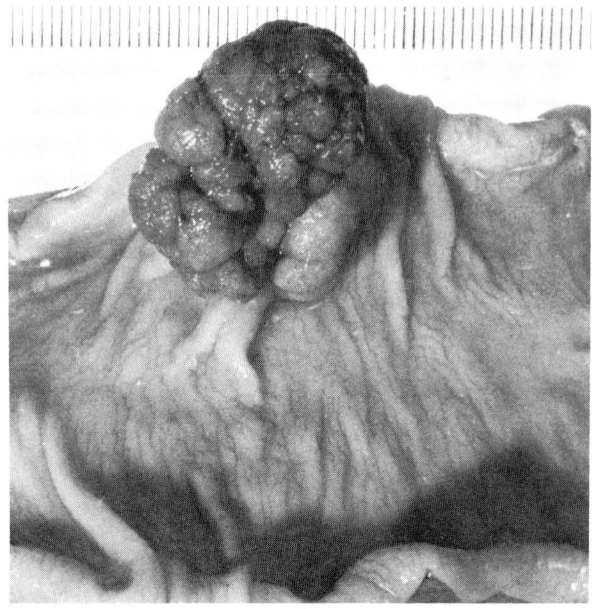

Figure 5–1 A 3-cm diameter pedunculated tubular adenoma.

(Fig. 5–2). However, tubular adenomas may be large and sessile, and a small pedunculated lesion can have a typical villous configuration. Careful inspection of the surface of many of these tumors can show a mixture of smooth and villous areas, or alternatively an intermediate or transitional type of morphology may be present (Fig. 5–3). The categorization of the macroscopic appearance of adenomas is important, since it may influence surgical treatment. Villous tumors, particularly when they are sessile, usually have a less circumscribed field of origin and a less defined edge than the tubular adenoma, and thus have a greater tendency to recur after local excision (Southwood, 1962). Adenomas, because of their vascularity and sometimes because of hemorrhage into them, secondary to trauma, are darker than the surrounding normal mucosa, although in small tumors this may not be very marked.

Microscopically, tubular adenomas consist of closely packed epithelial tubules, separated by normal lamina propria, which grow and branch horizontally to the muscularis mucosae (Fig. 5–4). The tubules can have a regular, well-differentiated structure or may show considerable irregularity, with much branching. There may be focal cystic dilatation of tubules, and secondary infection and hemorrhage may be

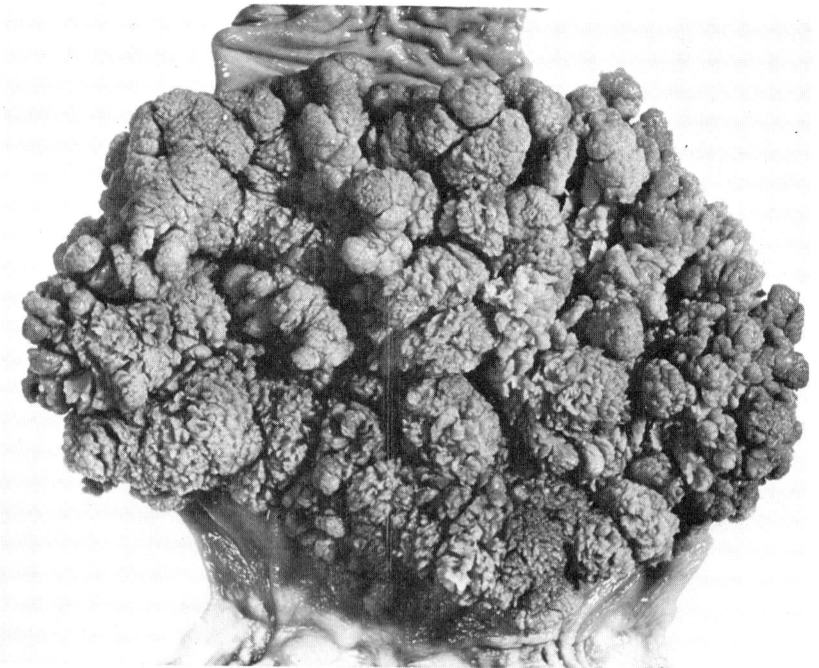

Figure 5–2 A huge sessile villous adenoma up to 15 cm in maximum dimension, which completely encircles the bowel wall.

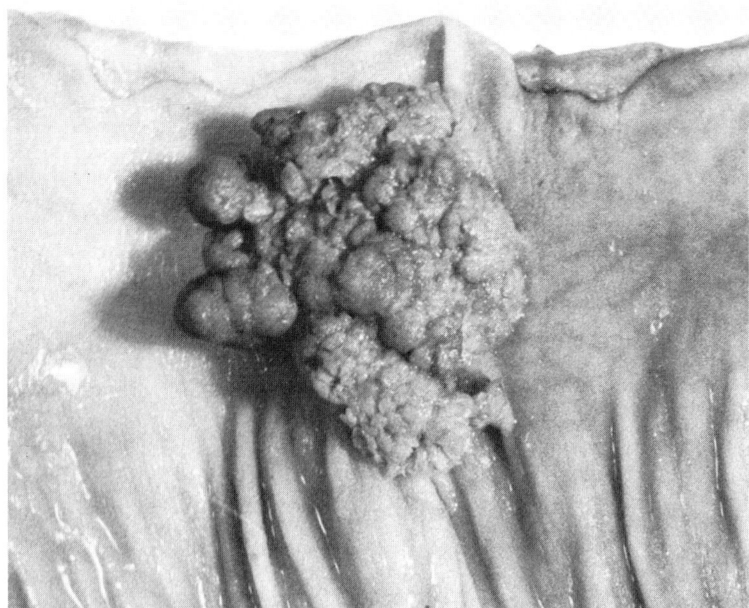

Figure 5–3 A 4-cm diameter tumor showing a mixture of smooth and villous areas, with the microscopic features of a tubulovillous adenoma.

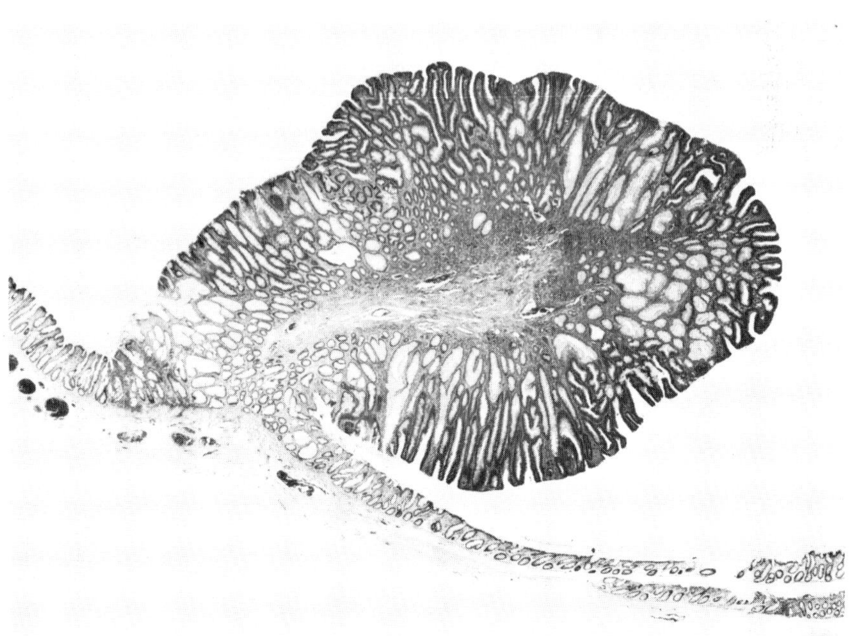

Figure 5–4 A pedunculated tubular adenoma. H&E × 11.

present in the substance of the tumor. The stalk of a pedunculated adenoma is composed of normal mucosa and submucosa. The villous adenoma consists of finger-like processes, each made up of a core of lamina propria covered by epithelial cells, growing vertically toward the bowel lumen. In between the processes, the epithelium rests on the muscularis mucosae (Fig. 5–5). Intermediate varieties of adenoma (tubulovillous) either can show a mixture of the tubular and villous patterns described above or, more commonly, can have a uniform histology with broad and stunted villi, deep to which are epithelial tubules similar to those in a tubular adenoma (Fig. 5–6).

The cytology of adenomas is similar irrespective of their histologic growth pattern. The nuclei are hyperchromatic and increased in number, resulting in a crowded appearance within the epithelium, and they occupy more of the cell than in normal mucosa. Increased numbers of mitoses are present throughout the tumor. Compared with normal the amount of mucus is sharply reduced, although in some villous adenomas, and exceptionally in tubular adenomas, it may be increased.

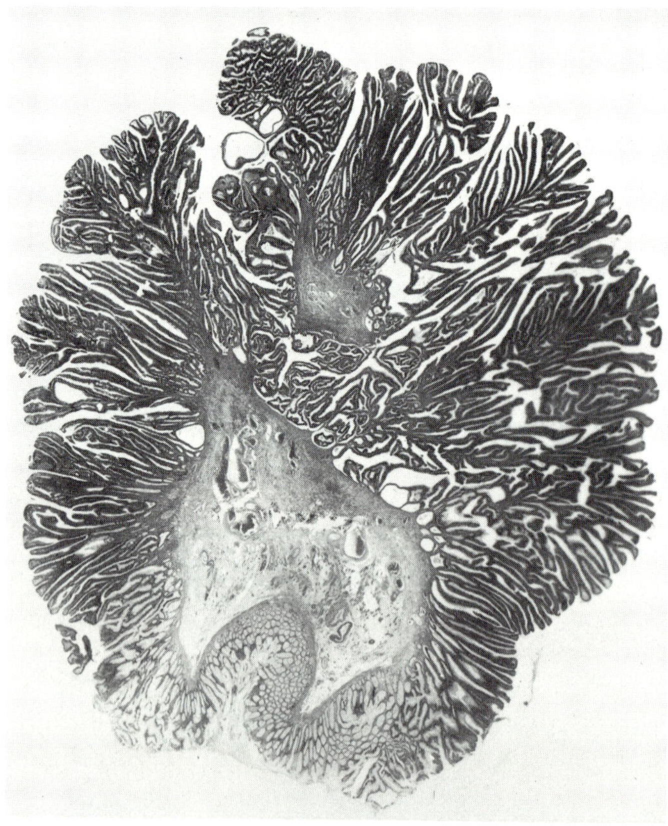

Figure 5–5 A 1.5-cm diameter villous adenoma. H&E × 6.

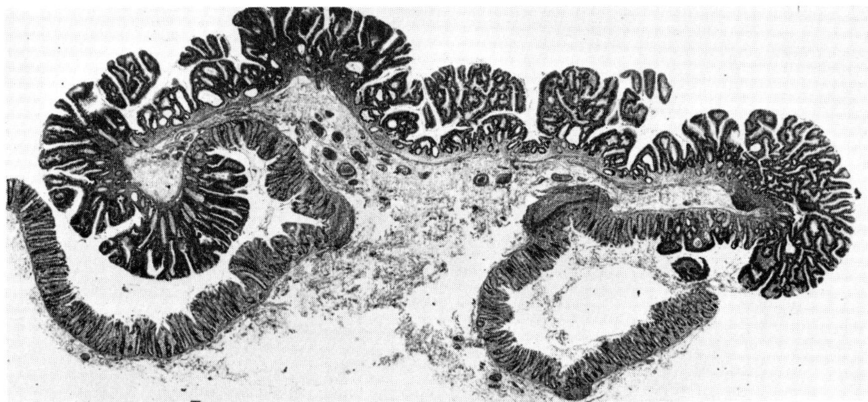

Figure 5–6 A sessile tubulovillous adenoma with a histologic pattern intermediate between that of a tubular and a villous adenoma. H&E × 14.5.

Atypia of nuclei is very common in all histologic types of adenomas, and varies in severity not only in different tumors but also within the same tumor. Atypia or dysplasia can be graded as mild, moderate, or severe on the basis of nuclear changes such as enlargement, pleomorphism, loss of polarity, stratification, and an increase in the number of mitotic figures, some of which may be abnormal forms (Fig. 5–7). Grading in this way is subjective and necessarily imprecise, since it is obvious that all gradations of dysplasia exist without the steplike transformations implicit in such a classification. Severe dysplasia has been equated by some histopathologists with carcinoma in situ, but the use of the latter expression in the diagnosis of tumors of the colon and rectum is best avoided as it is liable to misinterpretation by clinicians, with the attendant risk of unnecessarily radical surgery. With severe grades of dysplasia, as well as nuclear abnormalities, there is often distortion of the growth pattern of the glands with irregular budding and cribriform areas.

Although of limited practical significance in the description of the individual tumor, grading has been used to provide indirect evidence for the adenoma-carcinoma sequence (see Chapter 6).

Both Paneth and enterochromaffin cells may be scattered in a random manner throughout adenomas, and this can be a helpful feature in distinguishing them from non-neoplastic polyps such as the juvenile, Peutz-Jeghers, and metaplastic types in which, if present, these cells are situated at the base of the crypts.

CELL TURNOVER STUDIES

Using autoradiographic techniques based on the incorporation of tritium-labeled thymidine by cells synthesizing deoxyribonucleic acid

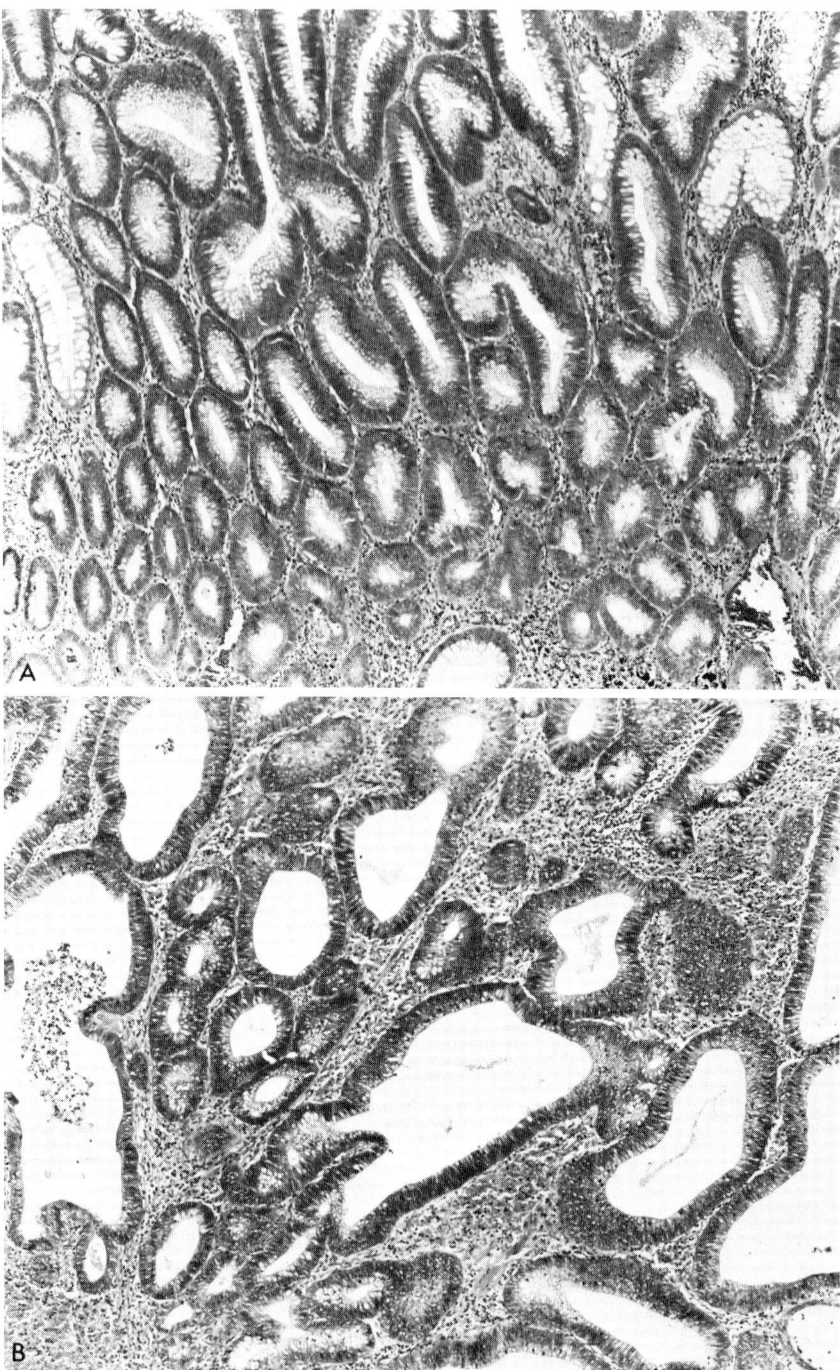

Figure 5–7 Degree of epithelial atypia in adenomas: *A*, mild; *B*, moderate; *C*, severe. H&E, all × 60.

Illustration continued on the opposite page

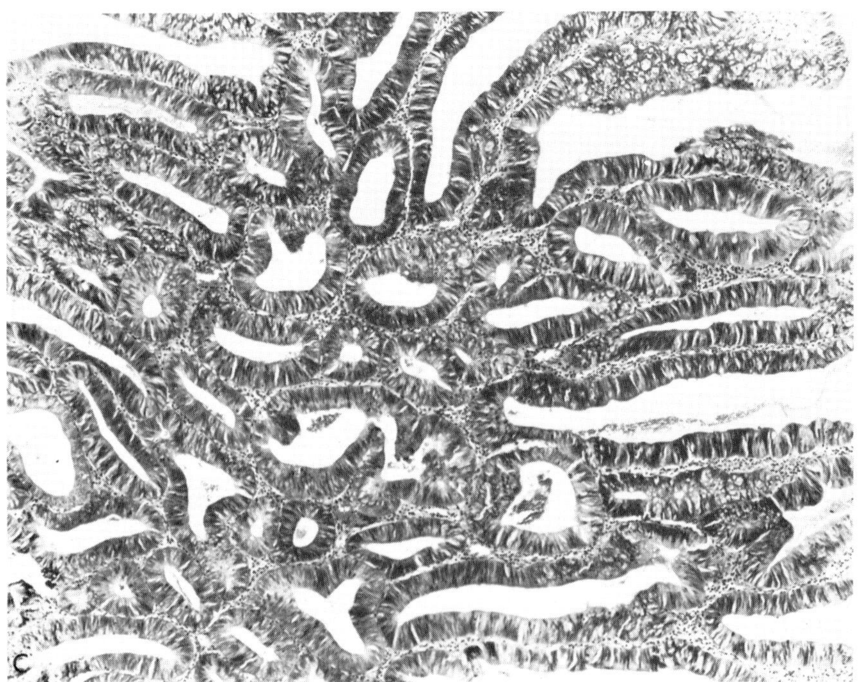

Figure 5–7 *Continued.*

(DNA), it has been possible to assess cell renewal in colonic mucosa in vivo. Thus it has been shown that the surface epithelium of colonic mucosa in a healthy person is replaced by new cells every four to eight days (Cole & McKalen, 1961; Lipkin et al., 1963; MacDonald et al., 1964). After rapid intravenous injection of tritiated thymidine, radioautographs on serial rectal biopsies show initial incorporation of the radioactively labeled substance into the nuclei at the bases of the crypts of Lieberkühn, and in successive specimens the labeled nuclei appear at progressively higher levels of the crypt, so that in a nine-day biopsy numerous labeled cells are present in the surface epithelium. In the normal colorectal mucosa, cell division is restricted to the lower third of the crypts, after which the cells move upward into the transitional zone, where DNA synthesis and mitosis stops and differentiation to mature goblet and absorptive cells occurs. Cell division and migration is perfectly balanced by exfoliation of cells from the surface mucosa. Lipkin (1974) and others have studied cell turnover in the colon of patients who have isolated adenomas or carcinomas, and in those patients with familial polyposis. They observed two types of change in some areas of histologically normal mucosa, which from animal experiments suggested that they were two sequential phases in the development of abnormal differentiation of colonic cells. In phase I some cells continued to incorporate thymidine into DNA during their migration to the surface of the mucosa, although there was no over-all increase in colonic cell population. In phase II, in addition to nonrepression of DNA synthesis, cells also develop properties that enable them to be retained in the colonic mucosa, so that a net increase in the number of cells occurs. It is the retention of these abnormally proliferating epithelial cells which is thought to give rise to adenomas.

HISTOCHEMISTRY

Histochemical studies of the enzyme content and pattern of mucosubstances in adenomas have shown features that distinguish them from normal mucosa, carcinoma, and other types of polyp. In a study of five oxidative enzymes in normal colon, metaplastic polyps, adenomas, and carcinomas (Wattenberg, 1959), a distinctive pattern was present in carcinomas, with high nicotinamide adenine dinucleotide (NAD) and nicotinamide adenine dinucleotide phosphate (NADP) activity, and low succinic dehydrogenase, α-glycerolphosphate dehydrogenase, and monoamine oxidase activity. In metaplastic polyps there was weak staining for succinic dehydrogenase, α-glycerolphosphate dehydrogenase, and monoamine oxidase, and although high NADP activity could occur, NAD activity was not increased. Adenomas showed a variable pattern, but a striking feature was intense staining for succinic dehydrogenase, α-glycerolphosphate dehydrogenase, and monoamine oxidase. Czernobilsky and Tsou (1968) found the enzyme pattern of inflammatory and juvenile polyps to be the same as in normal mucosa. In adenocarcinomas there was a loss of the hydrolytic enzymes acid phosphatase, esterase, and adenosine triphosphatase (ATPase), and diminished, but focally intense, activity of the respiratory enzyme succinic dehydrogenase. In "adenomatous" polyps there was a loss of hydrolytic enzymes but an increase in succinic dehydrogenase. Villous adenomas, atypical areas in adenomatous polyps, and hyperplastic polyps showed a diminution of all these enzymes.

Studies of mucosubstances have yielded interesting findings (Filipe, 1969; Filipe and Branfoot, 1974). In normal colonic mucosa, goblet cells secrete a mixture of sulfomucins and sialomucins, but their distribution throughout the crypt and along the surface epithelium varies. Thus in the deeper part of the crypt sulfomucins are more abundant, whereas in the upper half of the crypt both types of acid mucin are present. The surface epithelium also contains both types of mucin, but one or the other predominates. In adenomas the amount and type of mucus vary from zone to zone, but sulfomucins predominate. As they become less differentiated little or no mucus is formed; when present it consists mainly of sulfated mucins. In areas of malignant transformation, either no secretion or a scanty mixture of sulfated, nonsulfated, and neutral mucosubstances is found. Abnormal patterns of mucus secretion, with an increase in sialomucins and a decrease or absence of sulfomucins, is present in the mucosa adjacent to carcinomas and in patches away from them. This so-called transitional mucosa, which differs histochemically from the normal, has also been found adjacent to adenomas in cases of familial polyposis coli.

ULTRASTRUCTURE

A number of ultrastructural studies on both normal and adenomatous human colonic epithelium have been reported (Fisher and Sharkey, 1962; Imai et al., 1965; Pittman and Pittman, 1966; Lorenzsonn and Trier, 1968; Kavin et al., 1970; Kaye et al., 1973; Fenoglio et al., 1975). Kaye et al. (1973) compared the ultrastructural features of normal, hyperplastic, and adenomatous epithelium at three different levels of the crypt. In normal mucosa, four basic cell types were present: the undifferentiated, enterochromaffin, goblet, and absorptive cells. Ultrastructurally three kinds of partially differentiated cell, a so-called intermediate cell, and immature goblet and absorptive cells were seen. The last type of cell that could be identified was the hypermature or exhausted goblet cell. These eight cell types were found also in both hyperplastic and adenomatous lesions, but the relative ratios of mature to immature cells at each level of the crypt was different from the normal in each case. There was also an increase in the number of cells per crypt. Thus in normal mucosa a regular process of differentiation occurs from the base, where undifferentiated cells predominate, through intermediate cells and immature goblet and absorptive cells in the middle third, to the surface where the population is largely made up of mature absorptive cells and a few exhausted goblet cells. In hyperplastic mucosa there is an exaggeration of normal colonic differentiation, so that differentiated cells appear at lower levels of the crypt (see Chapter 2). In adenomas there is a failure of differentiation so that most cells in the upper third of the crypt and at the free surface are intermediate cells, and in some adenomas enterochromaffin cells are also present in this position.

In a study of tubular and villous adenomas (Imai et al., 1965) it was observed that focal disruptions of the basement membrane were present in the latter through which various amounts of cytoplasm protruded into the stroma. In tubular adenomas, the basement membrane was continuous. In villous adenomas the spaces between cells were wide, with short cytoplasmic processes from adjacent cells in contact with each other only focally, together with a lack of desmosomes. All these features, which were lacking in tubular adenomas, suggested decreased cell cohesiveness.

CHROMOSOMAL STUDIES

Observations on chromosomes in adenomas have been scanty. Messinetti et al. (1968) could find no numerical structural variation of chromosomes irrespective of epithelial atypia, but they described abnormalities in adenomas in which malignant change had occurred. In a study by Enterline and Arvan (1967) of 17 adenomas and seven carcinomas, variations in the number and structure of chromosomes were present even in adenomas without atypia. Thus, trisomy of one or more of the chromosomes was not uncommon, and the repetition of these changes in the same tumor led these authors to suggest that the adenoma could have originated through an initial chromosomal disjunction followed by perpetuation of the resulting trisomy. Pseudodiploid sets were common, but abnormal individual chromosomes uncommon, in adenomas without atypia; however, their frequency grew with increasing degree of atypia as did hyperploidy, which was marked in those adenomas with a villous component. Chromosome counts on adenocarcinomas showed a large number of cells in the triploid and tetraploid range. A gradation of chromosomal abnormalities, therefore, was seen from adenomas without atypia through to invasive carcinomas.

Similar observations have been made by Lubs and Kotler (1967), Baker and Atkin (1970), and Mark et al. (1973), the last-named authors noting in their material and from a study of the literature that variation in chromosome number most often involved groups C and D, other chromosome groups rarely being affected.

PSEUDOINVASION

The presence of benign adenomatous epithelium deep to the muscularis mucosae of adenomas has been described by several authors, although terminology has varied. Thus Fechner (1973) referred to this phenomenon as adenomatous polyp with submucosal cysts, Muto et al. (1973) as pseudocarcinomatous invasion, and Greene (1974) as epithelial misplacement in adenomatous polyps. Tangential sections through the irregular glandular base of an adenoma may artifactually produce the appearance of isolated islands of epithelium (Castleman and Krickstein, 1962), but in this case they are superficial to the muscularis mucosae.

In a study at St. Mark's Hospital (Muto et al., 1973) of 2,341 adenomas removed from 1,586 patients during the 12-year period 1957 to 1968, 56, or 2.4 per cent of the total, from 54 patients showed the criteria of pseudoinvasion. In the same period 110 adenomas, of tubular and villous types, had unequivocal evidence of invasive carcinoma into the submucosal layer only.

Histologic features of this condition are the presence of glandlike structures in the submucosa that show the same degree of dysplasia as the epithelium of the head of the adenoma, and are in continuity with it across the line of the muscularis mucosae (Fig. 5–8). The cytologic characteristics of malignancy are lacking. Submucosal glandular tissue is well-circumscribed, and individual glands are surrounded by lamina propria without the desmoplastic reaction to the epithelial cells that is usual in invasive carcinoma. In most cases (48 out of 56 adenomas in the St. Mark's series) deposits of hemosiderin pigment around the submucosal glands are present, and areas of recent hemorrhage are also common. Although hemosiderin is often seen in the head of typical adenomas, it is unusual in the underlying submucosa or in the neighborhood of early invasive carcinoma. Sometimes there is marked branching and excess of the muscularis mucosae.

Pseudoinvasion is particularly associated with larger tumors and in those with a long stalk, and is seen most commonly in adenomas of the sigmoid colon, the site of greatest muscular activity in the large bowel. Together with the histologic appearances, this suggests that the misplaced epithelium is secondary to hemorrhage due to repeated twisting of the stalk of the adenoma.

Follow-up studies on these patients have shown no evidence of recurrence or metastasis, confirming the benign behavior.

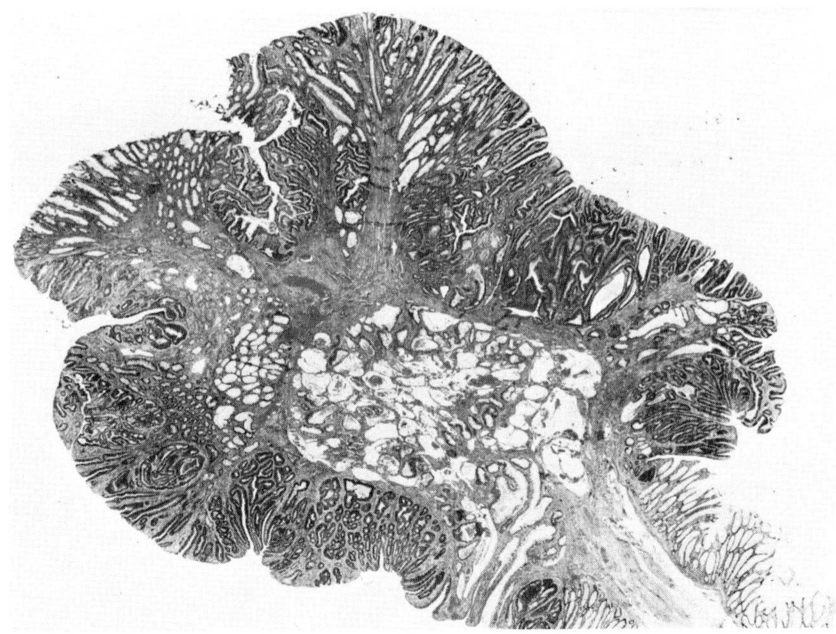

Figure 5–8 Pseudocarcinomatous invasion. Misplaced and cystically dilated glandular epithelium is present deep to the muscularis mucosae in the core of this otherwise typical tubular adenoma. H&E × 12.3.

The recognition of pseudoinvasion is important not only in the treatment of individual patients but also in the critical evaluation of the malignant transformation of adenomas.

References

Arminski, T. C., and McLean, D. W.: Incidence and distribution of adenomatous polyps of the colon and rectum based on 1,000 autopsy examinations. Dis. Colon Rectum *7*:249, 1964.

Baker, M. C., and Atkin, N. B.: Chromosome abnormalities in polyps and carcinomas of the large bowel. Proc. R. Soc. Med. (Suppl)*63*:9, 1970.

Blatt, L. J.: Polyps of the colon and rectum: incidence and distribution. Dis. Colon Rectum *4*:277, 1961.

Castleman, B., and Krickstein, H. I.: Do adenomatous polyps of the colon become malignant? N. Engl. J. Med. *267*:469, 1962.

Chapman, I.: Adenomatous polypi of large intestine: incidence and distribution. Ann. Surg. *157*:223, 1963.

Cole, J. W., and McKalen, A.: Observations of cell renewal in human rectal mucosa *in vivo* with thymidine–H^3. Gastroenterology *41*:122, 1961.

Czernobilsky, B., and Tsou, K-C.: Adenocarcinoma, adenomas and polyps of the colon. Histochemical study. Cancer *21*:165, 1968.

Enterline, H. T., and Arvan, D. A.: Chromosome constitution of adenoma and adenocarcinoma of the colon. Cancer *20*:1746, 1967.

Fechner, R. E.: Adenomatous polyp with submucosal cysts. Am. J. Clin. Pathol. *59*:498, 1973.

Fenoglio, C. M., Richart, R. M., and Kaye, G. I.: Comparative electron-microscopic features of normal, hyperplastic and adenomatous human colonic epithelium. II. Variations in surface architecture found by scanning electron microscopy. Gastroenterology *69*:100, 1975.

Filipe, M. I.: Value of histochemical reactions for mucosubstances in the diagnosis of certain pathological conditions of the colon and rectum. Gut *10*:577, 1969.

Filipe, M. I., and Branfoot, A. C.: Abnormal patterns of mucus secretion in apparently normal mucosa of large intestine with carcinoma. Cancer *34*:282, 1974.

Fisher, E. R., and Sharkey, D. A.: The ultrastructure of colonic polyps and cancer with special reference to the epithelial inclusion bodies of Leuchtenberger. Cancer *15*:160, 1962.

Greene, F. I.: Epithelial misplacement in adenomatous polyps of the colon and rectum. Cancer *33*:206, 1974.

Imai, H., Saito, S., and Stein, A. A.: Ultrastructure of adenomatous polyps and villous adenomas of the large intestine. Gastroenterology *48*:188, 1965.

Kavin, H., Hamilton, D. G., Greasley, R. E., Eckert, J. D., and Zuidema, G.: Scanning electron microscopy: a new method in the study of rectal mucosa. Gastroenterology *59*:426, 1970.

Kaye, G. I., Fenoglio, C. M., Pascal, R. R., and Lane, N.: Comparative electron microscopic features of normal, hyperplastic and adenomatous human colonic epithelium. Variations in cellular structure relative to the process of epithelial differentiation. Gastroenterology *64*:926, 1973.

Lipkin, M.: Phase I and phase II proliferative lesions of colonic epithelial cells in diseases leading to colonic cancer. Cancer *34*:878, 1974.

Lipkin, M., Bell, B., and Sherlock, P.: Cell proliferation kinetics in the gastrointestinal tract of man. I. Cell renewal in colon and rectum. J. Clin. Invest. *42*:767, 1963.

Lorenzsonn, V., and Trier, J. S.: The fine structure of human rectal mucosa. The epithelial lining of the base of the crypt. Gastroenterology *55*:88, 1968.

Lubs, H. A., and Kotler, S.: The prognostic significance of chromosome abnormalities in colon tumors. Ann. Intern. Med. *67*:328, 1967.

MacDonald, W. C., Trier, J. S., and Everett, N. B.: Cell proliferation and migration in the stomach, duodenum and rectum of man: radio-autographic studies. Gastroenterology *46*:405, 1964.

Mark, J., Mitelman, F., Dencker, H., Norryd, C., and Tranberg, K-G.: The specificity of the chromosomal abnormalities in human colonic polyps. A cytogenetic study of multiple polyps in a case of Gardner's syndrome. Acta Pathol. Microbiol. Scand. *81*:85, 1973.

Messinetti, S., Zelli, G. P., Marcellino, L. R., and Alcini, E.: Benign and malignant tumors of the gastrointestinal tract. Chromosome analysis in study and diagnosis. Cancer *21*:1000, 1968.

Muto, T., Bussey, H. J. R., and Morson, B. C.: Pseudo-carcinomatous invasion in adenomatous polyps of the colon and rectum. J. Clin. Pathol. *26*:25, 1973.

Pittman, F. E., and Pittman, J. C.: An electron microscopic study of the epithelium of normal human sigmoid colonic mucosa. Gut *7*:644, 1966.

Southwood, W. J. W.: Villous tumours of the large intestine. Ann. R. Coll. Surg. Engl. *30*:23, 1962.

Wattenberg, L. W.: A histochemical study of five oxidative enzymes in carcinoma of the large intestine in man. Am. J. Pathol. *35*:113, 1959.

Chapter Six

The Adenoma-Carcinoma Sequence

David W. Day and B. C. Morson

In this chapter adenomas as precancerous lesions, and the factors associated with malignant transformation of adenomas, will be discussed. Epidemiologic and experimental work relating to the adenoma-carcinoma sequence is considered later (see Chapters 10 and 11).

ADENOMA-CARCINOMA SEQUENCE

The evidence that adenomas can develop into carcinomas has been obtained from a variety of sources, some circumstantial and others more direct. First, about one in three of all operation specimens for cancer of the colon and rectum contain one or more adenomas (Morson and Dawson, 1972). That this is not merely coincidental is suggested by the fact that approximately 7 per cent of the group with one or more adenomas in addition to the carcinoma in the resected part of large bowel will develop a second or metachronous tumor in the remaining bowel; this is about twice the rate in the group of patients in which no associated adenomas are present (Bussey, Wallace, and Morson, 1967).

Second, in a series of 157 patients with synchronous carcinomas, i.e., two or more cancers found at the same time, and excluding patients with tumors associated with familial polyposis coli or ulcerative colitis, 75 per cent had associated adenomas (Heald and Bussey, 1975). Thus the concurrence of adenomas and carcinomas is not a chance event.

More direct evidence for the adenoma-carcinoma sequence comes from the finding of contiguous benign tumor in a carcinoma. Careful histologic study of malignant tumors thus may show all gradations from the adenoma with a microscopic focus of invasive adenocarcinoma (here defined as malignant tumor deep to the muscularis mucosae) to the obvious cancer with some residual benign tumor at one edge (Figs. 6–1 and 6–2). On occasion it is obvious from macroscopic inspection that the tumor is partly benign and partly malignant (Fig. 6–3). Sometimes what appears to be a benign tumor grossly is seen on microscopic examination to consist exclusively of adenocarcinoma (the so-called polypoid carcinoma – Fig. 6–4), and in these circumstances it is not possible to say whether the cancer arose from a previously benign adenoma. In a series of malignant tumors examined at St. Mark's Hospital between 1957 and 1968, 278 out of 1961 (14.2 per cent) contained varying proportions of adenomatous tissue (Muto, Bussey, and Morson, 1975). In these 'mixed' tumors, the benign component had the histologic structure of a tubular adenoma in 32.7 per cent of cases, of a tubulovillous adenoma in 31.3 per cent, and of a villous adenoma in 36.0 per cent; i.e., the histologic variants of adenomas were equally represented. Since approximately 75 per cent of adenomas unassociated with cancer have a tubular pattern, 15 per cent a tubulovillous, and 10 per cent a villous structure (these figures being obtained by the same observers), it follows that the villous type of growth has the higher malignant potential, and this will be alluded to later.

Further support for the adenoma-carcinoma sequence comes from

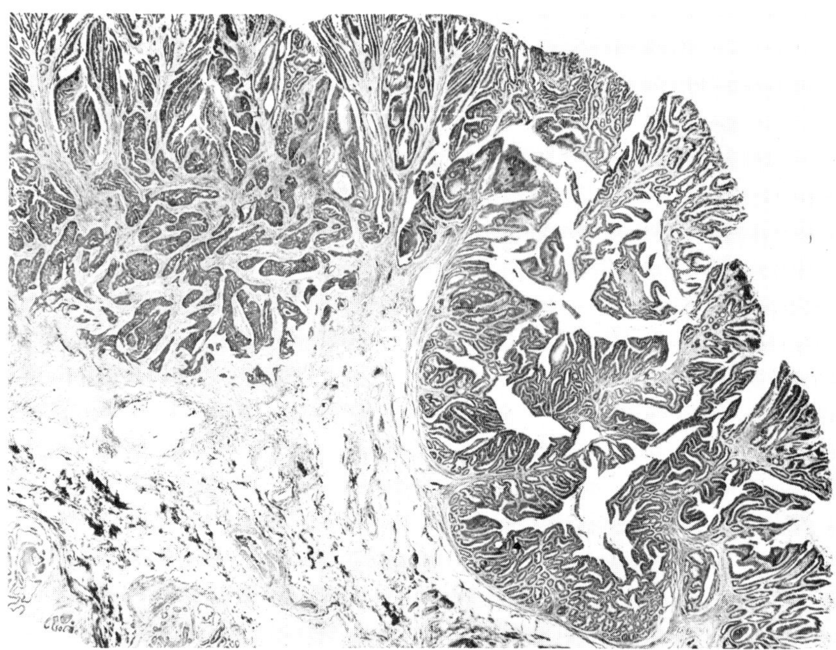

Figure 6–1 A focus of invasive adenocarcinoma arising in the head of a tubulovillous adenoma. H&E × 10.

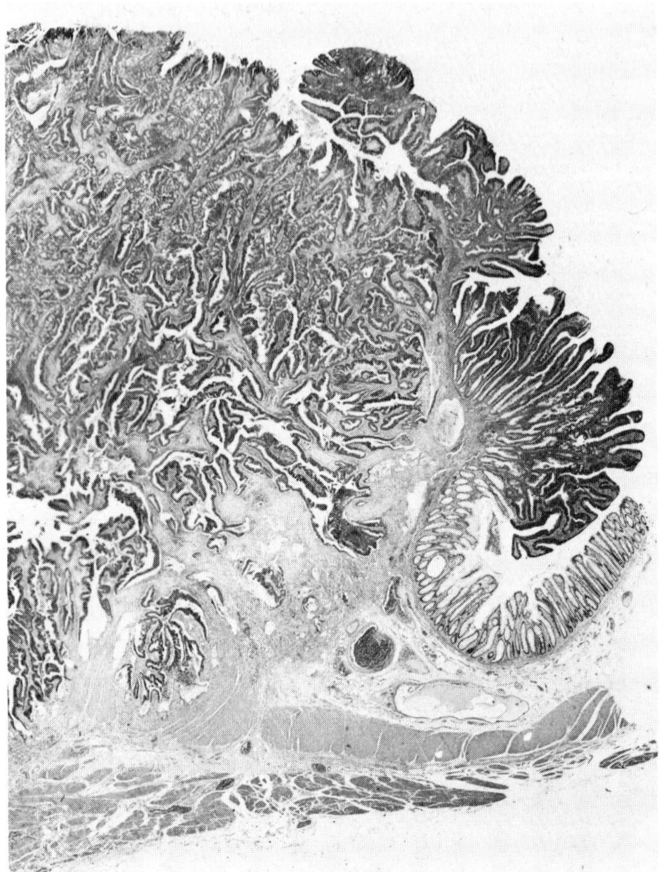

Figure 6–2 Residual adenomatous tissue at the edge of an invasive adenocarcinoma. H&E × 8.

a different series (Morson, 1966) in which the incidence of a benign component of large bowel carcinoma was related to the extent of spread of the tumor through the bowel wall. Benign tumor contiguous to the adenocarcinoma was found in only 7 per cent of cases in which there had been spread through the bowel wall to extramural fat; however, when spread was limited to the bowel wall an adenomatous component was observed in 20 per cent of cases, and with invasion only of the submucosal layer 60 per cent of cases contained some adenomatous tissue. These findings suggest that as a carcinoma enlarges, progressively more of the precursor adenoma is destroyed by or is transformed into malignant tissue. It would also seem from this study that most cancers of the colon and rectum arise from previously benign adenomas.

In the Heald and Bussey series of synchronous malignant tumors referred to above, of 323 cancers examined, 87 (27 per cent of the total) showed evidence of benign tumor adjacent to the invasive cancer.

If adenomas precede carcinomas, they would be expected to occur in a younger age-group. In familial polyposis coli in which hundreds or thousands of adenomas are present, one or more carcinomas invariably develop if operation is delayed. In this condition a clear difference occurs between the age at which polyps appear and the development of carcinoma in those patients who either refused operation or who had been treated by limited resection, leaving most of the colon still with polyps. However, leaving aside familial polyposis, surgical series comparing the ages of patients with adenomas and carcinomas have shown no difference (Grinnell and Lane, 1958; Enterline et al., 1962); this is most probably due to the fact that whereas the age at diagnosis of cancer may be fairly accurate, the age at diagnosis of an adenoma is likely to be very approximate because it usually does not give rise to symptoms. Figures from cancer detection clinics, where asymptomatic individuals are examined, do show a difference, however, with average

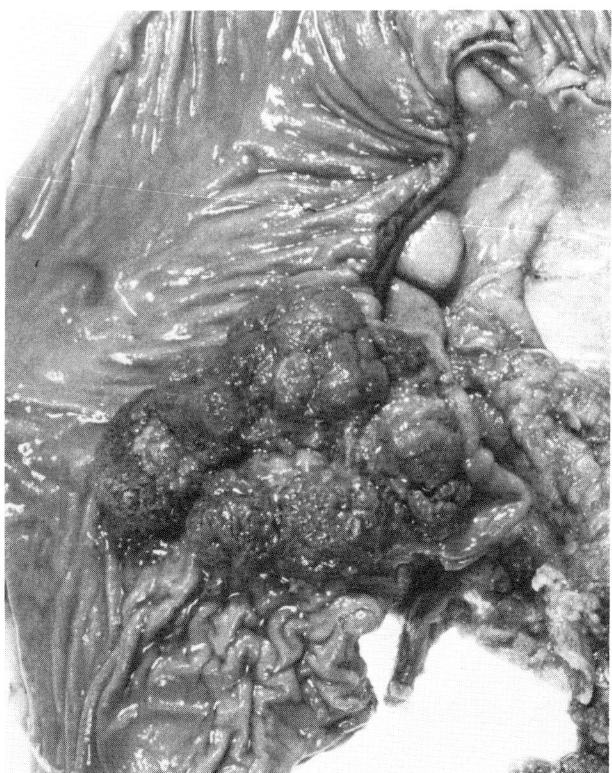

Figure 6–3 A 5-cm diameter villous tumor in which invasive carcinoma arises in the central ulcerated zone.

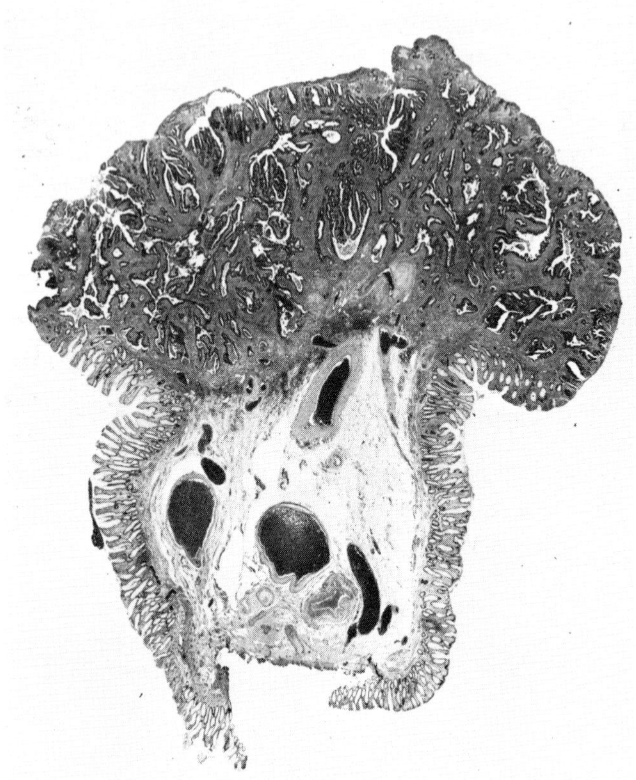

Figure 6–4 Polypoid carcinoma. No residual adenomatous tissue is present. H&E × 10.

ages of 50.2 years for adenoma and 57.6 years for carcinoma (Enterline, 1976).

What about the distribution of adenomas and carcinomas? In the previous chapter the problems associated with determining the site distribution of adenomas were discussed in an attempt to explain the discrepancies between different published series. For obvious reasons the distribution of carcinomas in the large bowel is easier to ascertain, and as a result there is much better correlation between different reports. As a representative example, Falterman et al. (1974), analyzing their 2,313 cases of cancer of the large bowel, found that 18 per cent occurred in the cecum and ascending colon, 9 per cent in the transverse colon, 7 per cent in the descending colon, and 65 per cent in the sigmoid and rectum. Ekelund (1963) conducted an extensive study of colorectal adenomas and carcinomas in the population of Malmö, Sweden. Of the 60 per cent of the population who died in hospital the autopsy rate was approximately 99 per cent. In the 3,398 cases autopsied in a three-year period, adenomas were found in 25.6 per cent of patients with cancer and in 11 per cent of those without. The distribution of solitary adenomas was similar to that of carcinomas, 56.1 per cent of the adenomas being in the sigmoid and rectum compared to 63.3 per cent of carcinomas at the same sites, and 18.8 per cent of the adenomas being in the cecum and ascending colon compared to 21 per cent of carcinomas. When both solitary and multiple adenomas were considered, the distribution was relatively more even throughout the large bowel than that of carcinoma. Thus an approximate, but not exact, association exists between the sites of adenoma and carcinoma, with some excess of adenomas in the right colon and some deficit of adenomas in the sigmoid colon and rectum.

The studies of Spratt and co-workers (1958) on patients with both adenomas and carcinomas in the same resection specimen showed that adenomas tended to be more distal to the carcinoma in the cecum and ascending colon, and more proximal in the sigmoid and rectum. They proposed that if adenomas give rise to carcinomas, the distribution of adenomas in such cases should be randomly distributed in relation to the carcinomas, with equal numbers proximal and distal to the malignancy. However, this assumes that adenomas have an equal propensity for malignant change irrespective of their site.

MALIGNANT POTENTIAL

Evidence has been presented to show that adenomas may progress to carcinomas, but in view of the disproportionate prevalence of adenomas compared with adenocarcinomas in western populations it is obvious that malignant transformation is a relatively uncommon event. What then determines the malignant potential of adenomas? Three factors, probably interrelated, which have been shown to be important are the size, the growth pattern, and the degree of epithelial atypia of adenomas.

Size

Several studies have shown that the malignant potential is increased in large adenomas compared with small adenomas (Grinnell and Lane, 1958; Enterline et al., 1962; Silverberg, 1970). Grinnell and Lane divided their series of 1,856 adenomas into four groups: benign adenomatous polyps (tubular adenomas) and papillary adenomas (villous adenomas), with and without secondary invasive cancer. The average diameter of benign adenomatous polyps was 1.2 cm and of papillary adenomas 3.7 cm, but in those with associated carcinoma the diameters were 2.1 and 4.2 cm respectively. Of the 47 adenomatous polyps with invasive cancer, only one had a diameter of less than 0.5 cm, and only three were between 0.5 and 1.0 cm in diameter; this represents a rate of 0.3 and 0.9 per cent respectively out of the total of 1,352 adenomatous polyps with reported measurements. By contrast the malignancy rate rose to 9.3 per cent in those lesions in the 1.5-, to 2.5-cm size range, and to more than 12 per cent in those 2.5 cm in diameter or greater. Although the rate of increase was less striking the same trend was noted with papillary adenomas.

The experience at St. Mark's Hospital (Morson, 1974) shows that the prevalence of cancer in adenomas under 1 cm in size is only about 1 per cent; in those between 1 and 2 cm in diameter it is about 10 per cent; and in those over 2 cm there is a nearly 50 per cent malignancy rate. Table 6–1 shows that about 60 per cent of all the polyps in this series were small (under 1 cm in diameter), about 20 to 25 per cent were 1 to 2 cm in size, and only 15 to 20 per cent were over 2 cm in diameter. This suggests that as adenomas grow, and there is direct evidence that they can (Mayo and de Castro, 1956; Scarborough, 1960; Linnell et al., 1963; Figiel et al., 1965; Smith et al., 1970), so the cancer risk rises. However, taking into account the difference in prevalence between adenomas and carcinomas, it follows that most adenomas do not grow appreciably and may never reach sufficient size to become significantly at risk from malignant change.

Histologic Type

The classification of adenomas into those with a predominantly tubular pattern, those with a mainly villous pattern, and those with either a mixture of tubular and villous areas or with an intermediate type of histology has shown that in general the adenoma with a villous pattern has a higher malignant potential than one with a tubular pattern. Thus, in the St. Mark's material, the malignancy rate for tubular adenomas is about 5 per cent but rises to 40 per cent in villous adenomas. The rate for the intermediate or tubulovillous type (22 per cent) suggests that these tumors behave more like villous than tubular adenomas. The subdivision of adenomas on the basis of their growth pattern, as well as being subjective, is also dependent on sampling. Fung and Goldman (1970) in a retrospective histologic review of adenomas found focal villous change in 6 per cent of solitary tumors, but in a

TABLE 6–1 The Size of Adenomas in Relation to Malignancy Rate

Size of Tumor	Total Number	Number with Malignancy	Percentage
Under 1 cm	1,479	19	1.3
1–2 cm	580	55	9.5
Over 2 cm	430	198	46.0

TABLE 6–2 Relationship of Size and Histologic Type of Tumor

Type of Tumor	Under 1 cm	1–2 cm	Over 2 cm
Tubular adenoma	76.6%	19.7%	3.7%
Intermediate type	24.7%	46.8%	28.5%
Villous adenoma	14.0%	25.7%	60.3%

prospective study using a dissecting microscope and multiple histologic sections this figure rose to 35 per cent, reaching 75 per cent in solitary lesions larger than 1 cm in diameter. The frequency with which a villous growth pattern is found increases with the size of the tumor (Table 6–2), and this points to the possibility that as adenomas grow there is an increasing tendency for them to adopt a villous type of structure (Kaneko, 1972). However, small pedunculated villous tumors and large sessile adenomatous polyps are seen. The growth pattern of adenomas is probably related to the size of the field of origin of a tumor as well as other more dynamic factors. In Table 6–3 the malignant potential of adenomas has been calculated on the basis of their size and histologic type. This shows that the very common tubular adenoma under 1 cm in diameter has a very low malignant potential (1 per cent), whereas the small villous tumor, which is rare, has a 10 per cent malignancy rate. The intermediate histologic type, also rarely this size, has a malignant potential of about 4 per cent. In those tumors between 1 and 2 cm in diameter there is no significant variation in the malignancy rate with histologic type, but with polyps over 2 cm in diameter the malignant potential is significantly greater for tumors with a villous component than for adenomatous polyps.

Whereas nobody has denied that villous tumors may and often do develop malignant change, the controversy has centered around adenomatous polyps (tubular adenomas); some authors state that these invariably become malignant, and others maintain that they never or very rarely do so (see, for example, Spratt et al., 1958; Helwig, 1959; Castleman and Krickstein, 1962; Lescher et al., 1967). The recognition of a spectrum of histologic appearances, and the appreciation of the importance of size in the malignant potential of adenomas, make much of this argument redundant.

TABLE 6–3 Adenomas: Percentage of Carcinoma in Relation to Size and Histologic Type

Histologic Type	Under 1 cm	1–2 cm	Over 2 cm
Tubular adenoma	1.0% (1,382)	10.2% (392)	34.7% (101)
Intermediate type	3.9% (76)	7.4% (149)	45.8% (155)
Villous adenoma	9.5% (21)	10.3% (39)	52.9% (174)

Although histologic type is very important in the assessment of malignant potential, it does seem that size has the paramount place (Enterline et al., 1962). One reason why villous tumors have a much greater cancer rate than adenomatous polyps could just be that they are usually much larger tumors. However, a study of the cytologic appearances in the three histologic types of polyp emphasizes the importance of the degree of epithelial atypia, and explains why even small villous tumors have a ten times greater malignant potential than adenomatous polyps of the same size.

Epithelial Atypia

The grading of adenomas into those showing mild, moderate, or severe dysplasia (see the previous chapter) has shown that, irrespective of histologic growth pattern, their malignant potential increases with increasing degrees of atypia. The severity of atypia is also related to the size of the tumor. From Table 6–4 it can be seen that small adenomas under 1 cm in diameter, which make up the majority of tumors in this study, usually show mild atypia only and have a very low malignant potential. The malignancy rate rises to 27 per cent if severe atypia is present, but this is very rare in a polyp of this size. A similar relationship is seen in polyps 1 to 2 cm in diameter; those with mild atypia have a low malignant potential, whereas those with moderate and severe atypia are increasingly likely to contain invasive foci. In adenomas over 2 cm in size the malignancy rate is high but shows little relation to the degree of atypia. This could be due to sampling error, but it also shows again how, in practice, size is of major importance in the assessment of malignant potential. In Table 6–5 the cancer rates are charted according to the degree of atypia in the three histologic variants of adenoma. The explanation for the high malignant potential in tumors with a villous component and mild or moderate atypia could be partly explained by a sampling error in the study of this group. Larger adenomas often show variable atypia in different parts of the same tumor, and it is conceivable that the sections examined were not representative. It is also possible that sections of these larger tumors were taken from areas away from the malignant focus, which itself arose from a localized area of severe atypia.

TABLE 6–4 Adenomas: Percentage of Carcinoma in Relation to Size and Grade of Atypia

Grade of Atypia	Under 1 cm	1–2 cm	Over 2 cm
Mild	0.3% (1,198)	3.0% (329)	42.3% (196)
Moderate	2.0% (244)	14.4% (167)	50.0% (134)
Severe	27.0% (37)	24.1% (83)	48.0% (100)

TABLE 6–5 Adenomas: Percentage of Carcinoma in Relation to Grade of Atypia and Histologic Type

Grade of Atypia	Tubular Adenoma	Intermediate	Villous Adenoma
Mild	2.0% (1,410)	13.9% (208)	36.2% (116)
Moderate	8.7% (357)	31.9% (119)	41.1% (73)
Severe	27.4% (113)	33.9% (56)	50.0% (54)

The demonstration of grades of epithelial atypia in adenomas is powerful support for the concept of the adenoma-carcinoma sequence (Lescher et al., 1967; Potet and Soullard, 1971; Kozuka, 1975), and suggests a gradual transition from a benign to a malignant tumor. It is probable that all carcinomas arising from epithelial surfaces have passed through stages of increasingly severe epithelial atypia before becoming invasive, and in the colon and rectum such a progression is seen only in adenomatous polyps and villous adenomas. At any rate, no alternative mechanism for the histogenesis of large bowel carcinoma has yet been documented (Fenoglio and Lane, 1974; Muto et al., 1975). Thus, small areas of severe dysplasia other than those arising in long-standing ulcerative colitis (Morson and Pang, 1967; Riddell, 1976) have not been observed independent of adenomas, nor have very small invasive carcinomas without ulceration been seen. Small ulcerated invasive cancers without residual adenomatous tissue have been described (Weingarten and Turell, 1952; Spratt and Ackerman, 1962), but these could result from continued invasion plus surface ulceration in an adenoma, so that all adenomatous remnants and indeed the stalk, if present, would disappear, leaving an ulcerated plaque of carcinoma bordered by nonadenomatous mucosal epithelium. This course of events would be more likely in the case of tubular and tubulovillous adenomas, especially those on pedicles in the presence of advanced cancer, than it would in the typical broad-based sessile villous adenoma, which would logically be expected to retain adenomatous elements even with advanced invasive cancer (Enterline, 1976).

If carcinoma did arise on a background of normal mucosa, numerous examples of tiny independent carcinomas under 0.5 cm in diameter would have been encountered and reported. That this is not the case is strong presumptive evidence against a de novo origin of large bowel cancer.

LIFE HISTORY

Given that adenomas under certain circumstances may develop malignant change, how long does it take for this to occur? In practice opportunities to follow this transition are very infrequent, since the usual treatment when a "polyp" is seen is its prompt removal. However, observations on this sequence have been made in two clinical situations: first, in a small number of patients who have had a benign tumor and refused operation or failed to re-attend after initial diagnosis, and who subsequently developed a carcinoma at the same site; and second, on patients with familial polyposis coli.

The first group includes four patients in the records of St. Mark's Hospital with adenomatous polyps of the rectum (Fig. 6–5). Patient 1 had a clinically benign adenomatous polyp, and five years three months after its detection presented with a carcinoma at the same site, which when resected showed a well-differentiated adenocarcinoma with residual benign adenomatous tissue at its edge. In the second patient there was a six-year interval between the clinical and biopsy diagnosis of adenomatous polyp and the detection of a carcinoma, and in patient 3 there was a 13-year interval between the observation of a polyp and the diagnosis of cancer. Patient 4 had a typical benign adenomatous polyp diagnosed histologically which was known to be present for over 11 years before its removal. Studies on patients with villous adenomas treated by repeated local excision or fulguration have shown that the tumors may remain histologically benign for many years. In two cases in which malignant change eventually developed, benign tumor had been observed for 10 years and nearly 30 years respectively (Morson, 1974).

Observations such as these are useful in that they confirm that adenomas may never develop malignant change, and in those that do the sequence evolves over a long period, although it probably is extremely variable. Together with studies of metachronous cancer rates and age distribution curves, they suggest that the adenoma-carcinoma

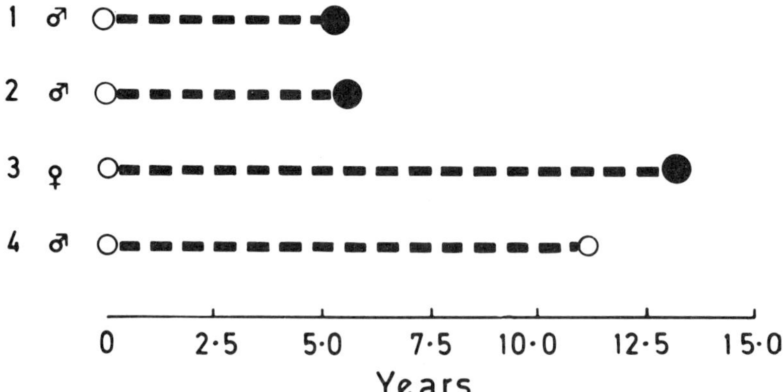

Figure 6–5 Fate of four untreated adenomatous polyps.

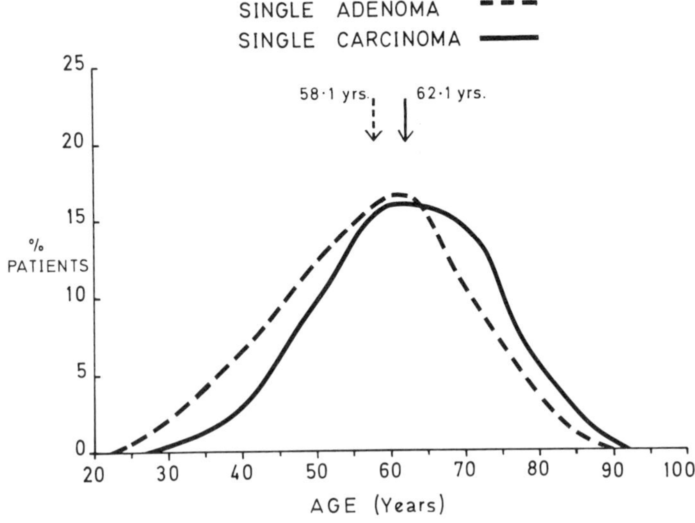

Figure 6–6 Age distribution for polyposis and cancer.

sequence is never less than five years, and averages 10 to 15 years, but may even cover a normal adult life span.

In patients with familial polyposis coli, the age distribution curves show a time interval of about 12 years between the average age at diagnosis of polyposis without cancer and of polyposis with cancer (Fig. 6–6). This difference is likely to be an underestimate since determination of the age at onset of polyposis is inaccurate, although probably less so than for isolated adenomas. More information on the life history comes from an analysis of the time of onset of polyposis and cancer in patients with familial polyposis coli who were not operated on. Most of these patients come from the group who were under care at St. Mark's Hospital before the operation of total colectomy and ileorectal anastomosis was established about 30 years ago. In Table 6–6 it can be

TABLE 6–6 Length of the Precancerous Phase in Familial Polyposis Coli

Period (Years)	Number of Patients Observed	Number Surviving Period Without Cancer	Number Developing Cancer in Period	Percentage Developing Cancer
0–5	65	59	6	9.2
5–10	45	35	10	22.2
10–15	23	16	7	30.4
15–20	12	8	4	33.3
20–25	7	4	3	42.6
25–30	3	1	2	66.6
30–35	1	–	1	100.0

seen that in 65 patients who did not have an operation, the likelihood of a carcinoma developing rose progressively as the period of observation increased. However, in the group of seven patients observed for 20 to 25 years, four did not develop carcinoma and one patient survived over 30 years before a malignant tumor supervened.

SUMMARY

Evidence has been presented to show that most carcinomas of the large bowel develop in an adenoma, and that the life history of this sequence, although variable, probably takes on average 10 to 15 years. However, when the absolute numbers of adenomas and carcinomas are compared, it is apparent that the transition is uncommon. On a statistical analysis the malignant potential of adenomas is related to their size, growth pattern, and degree of epithelial atypia. If the adenoma-carcinoma sequence is the norm, then a study of these criteria in adenomas at different sites in the colon and rectum would resolve the disparity in published series between the distribution of adenomas and carcinomas.

References

Bussey, H. J. R., Wallace, M. H., and Morson, B. C.: Metachronous carcinoma of the large intestine and intestinal polyps. Proc. R. Soc. Med. *60*:208, 1967.

Castleman, B., and Krickstein, H. I.: Do adenomatous polyps of the colon become malignant? N. Engl. J. Med. *267*:469, 1962.

Ekelund, G.: On cancer and polyps of colon and rectum. Acta Pathol. Microbiol. Scand. *59*:165, 1963.

Enterline, H. T.: Polyps and Cancer of the Large Bowel. *In* Morson, B. C. (ed.): Current Topics in Pathology. Vol. 63 – Pathology of the Gastrointestinal Tract. Springer-Verlag, Berlin, pp. 95–141, 1976.

Enterline, H. T., Evans, G. W., Mercado-Lugo, R., Miller, L., and Fitts, W. T., Jr.: Malignant potential of adenomas of colon and rectum. J.A.M.A. *179*:322, 1962.

Falterman, K. W., Hill, C. B., Markey, J. C., Fox, J. W., and Cohn, I., Jr.: Cancer of the colon, rectum and anus: a review of 2313 cases. Cancer *34*:951, 1974.

Fenoglio, C. M., and Lane, N.: The anatomical precursor of colorectal carcinoma. Cancer *34*:819, 1974.

Figiel, L. S., Figiel, S. J., and Wietersen, F. K.: Roentgenologic observations of growth rates of colonic polyps and carcinoma. Acta Radiol. *3*:417, 1965.

Fung, C. H. K., and Goldman, H.: The incidence and significance of villous change in adenomatous polyps. Am. J. Clin. Pathol. *53*:21, 1970.

Grinnell, R. S., and Lane, N.: Benign and malignant adenomatous polyps and papillary adenomas of the colon and rectum. An analysis of 1856 tumors in 1335 patients. Surgery *106*:519, 1958.

Heald, R. J., and Bussey, H. J. R.: Clinical experiences at St. Mark's Hospital with multiple synchronous cancers of the colon and rectum. Dis. Colon Rectum *18*:6, 1975.

Helwig, E. B.: Adenomas and pathogenesis of cancer of colon and rectum. Dis. Colon Rectum *2*:5, 1959.

Horn, R. C., Jr.: Malignant potential of polypoid lesions of the colon and rectum. Cancer *28*:146, 1971.

Kaneko, M.: On pedunculated adenomatous polyps of colon and rectum with particular reference to their malignant potential. Mt. Sinai J. Med. *39*:103, 1972.

Kozuka, S.: Premalignancy of the mucosal polyp in the large intestine. I. Histologic gradation of the polyp on the basis of epithelial pseudostratification and glandular branching. Dis. Colon Rectum *18*:483, 1975.

Lescher, T. C., Dockerty, M. B., Jackman, R. J., and Beahrs, O. H.: Histopathology of the larger colonic polyp. Dis. Colon Rectum *10*:118, 1967.

Linnell, F., Spout, H. J., and Johnson, R. E.: The rates and patterns of growth of 375 tumors of the large intestine and rectum observed serially by double contrast enema study (Malmö technique). Am. J. Roentgenol. *90*:673, 1963.

Mayo, C. W., and de Castro, C. A.: Carcinoma of the sigmoid arising from a polyp first visualised 15 years previously: report of a case. Mayo Clin. Proc. *31*:597, 1956.

Morson, B. C.: Factors influencing the prognosis of early cancer of the rectum. Proc. R. Soc. Med. *59*:607, 1966.

Morson, B. C.: The polyp cancer sequence in the large bowel. Proc. R. Soc. Med. *67*:451, 1974.

Morson, B. C., and Dawson, I. M. P.: Gastrointestinal Pathology. Blackwell Scientific, Oxford, 1972.

Morson, B. C., and Pang, L.: Rectal biopsy as an aid to cancer control in ulcerative colitis. Gut *8*:423, 1967.

Muto, T., Bussey, H. J. R., and Morson, B. C.: The evolution of cancer of the colon and rectum. Cancer *36*:2251, 1975.

Potet, F., and Soullard, J.: Polyps of the rectum and colon. Gut *12*:468, 1971.

Riddell, R. H.: The Precarcinomatous Phase of Ulcerative Colitis. *In* Morson, B. C. (ed.): Current Topics in Pathology. Vol. 63—Pathology of the Gastrointestinal Tract. Springer-Verlag, Berlin, pp. 179–219, 1976.

Scarborough, R. A.: The relationship between polyps and carcinoma of the colon and rectum. Dis. Colon Rectum *3*:336, 1960.

Silverberg, S. G.: Focally malignant adenomatous polyps of the colon and rectum. Surg. Gynecol. Obstet. *131*:103, 1970.

Smith, T. R., Maeir, D. M., Metcalf, W., and Kaplowitz, I. S.: Transformation of a pedunculated colonic polyp to adenocarcinoma? Dis. Colon Rectum *13*:382, 1970.

Spratt, J. S., Jr., and Ackerman, L. V.: Small primary adenocarcinomas of the colon and rectum. J.A.M.A. *179*:337, 1962.

Spratt, J. S., Jr., Ackerman, L. V., and Moyer, C. A.: Relationship of polyps of colon to colonic cancer. Ann. Surg. *148*:682, 1958.

Weingarten, M., and Turell, R.: Carcinomatous mucosal excrescence of the rectum. J.A.M.A. *149*:1467, 1952.

Chapter Seven

Multiple Adenomas and Carcinomas

H. J. R. Bussey

Any pathologist whose work involves the examination of surgical specimens from the large intestine is soon impressed by the frequency with which multiple tumors are found (Fig. 7–1). This perhaps is not surprising. Measuring some 150 cm in length and with an average surface area of at least 1,000 cm², all subject to genetic and environmental factors responsible for tumor formation, the human large intestine would seem an obvious site for multiple growths. Probably more tumors are found in the colon and rectum than in the rest

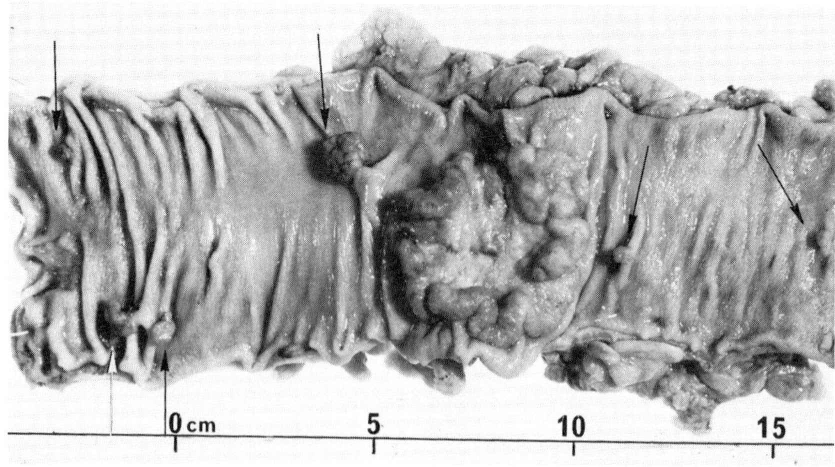

Figure 7–1 Portion of sigmoid colon resected for carcinoma. In addition to the malignant growth, at least six adenomatous polyps are present.

of the body. Not all of these are neoplastic, but adenomas and carcinomas are the most important.

FREQUENCY OF MULTIPLE TUMORS

A survey of patients seen at St. Mark's Hospital during the 12-year period 1957 to 1968 showed that there were 3,002 who had either adenomas or adenocarcinomas of the large intestine, or both. In 2,412 patients (80.3 per cent) only one tumor was found, 1,023 having an adenoma and 1,389 an adenocarcinoma. Multiple tumors, benign or malignant, were present synchronously in 590 patients (19.7 per cent). Thus, one in five of the patients with neoplastic disease of the large intestine had more than one tumor in the colon or rectum when first seen. Moreover, 146 (6.0 per cent) of the 2,412 patients who had a single tumor treated on the first occasion subsequently presented with one or more additional neoplasms of the large bowel, making the proportion of those known to have multiple tumors 736 out of 3,002, or 24.5 per cent (Table 7–1).

Since barium enema examinations were not carried out on all patients in whom only one intestinal tumor had been found, and since in many cases patients did not return for follow-up examinations, it is likely that the figure of 24.5 per cent for the incidence rate of multiple tumors is a considerable underestimate. Colonoscopy was not generally available during the period covered by the survey, and there is little doubt that its increased subsequent use will reveal a larger number of patients with multiple intestinal tumors.

The high incidence of multiple tumors in the large intestine has clinical implications that must influence the policy adopted when even a single tumor has been discovered in a patient. It is obvious that the

TABLE 7–1 Incidence of Multiple Tumors of the Large Intestine

St. Mark's Hospital, 1957–1968

Number of patients having initially		
1 adenoma only	1023	
1 carcinoma only	1389	
Total	2412	80.3%
Multiple adenomas or carcinomas	590	19.7%
Total	3002	
Number of patients with multiple synchronous adenomas or carcinomas initially	590	
Number of patients with solitary tumor initially who develop other tumors subsequently	146	
Total patients with multiple tumors	736	24.5%

whole large intestine must be investigated, either by barium enema examination or by colonoscopy, for other tumors that may be present simultaneously. Moreover, since there is a further risk of more tumors developing in the future, such examinations should be made at regular intervals. The available evidence indicates that, in general, adenomas grow slowly and require a period of several years before becoming a threat to the patient's well-being. Against this must be set the difficulty of being sure that the colon was completely free from all tumors at the previous examination. As a compromise it is suggested that the interval between examinations need not be less than three years and should not be more than five years, although these limits may have to be modified as more follow-up information is accumulated.

MULTIPLE ADENOMAS

Mention of multiple adenomas of the large intestine usually suggests the disease known as "familial polyposis coli," which is, of course, the ultimate in multiplicity of intestinal tumors and which is discussed in Chapter 8. However, multiple adenomas may be present in some patients who cannot be regarded as suffering from familial polyposis coli. It is therefore necessary to attempt a numerical distinction between the two groups of patients.

The survey of St. Mark's Hospital patients with intestinal neoplasms also revealed that there were 1,846 who had one or more adenomas, either wholly benign or with a focus of malignant change. An analysis into groups with varying numbers of adenomas per patient gave the results shown in Table 7–2. More than one-quarter of the patients had multiple adenomas. It has already been mentioned that these results were obtained from a period when colonoscopy had not been introduced. A further analysis in a few years' time would undoubtedly show an increase in the number of patients with two to five adenomas at the expense of those with only a solitary adenoma, usually discovered incidentally in patients presenting with symptoms due to other pathology. On the other hand, the presence of five or more adenomas, either synchronously or metachronously, usually means that the patient

TABLE 7–2 Frequency of Multiple Adenomas

No. of Adenomas	No. of Patients	Percentage
1	1,331	72.1
2–5	432	23.4
More than 5	83	4.5
TOTAL	1,846	100.0

has been subjected to repeated sigmoidoscopic examinations and barium enema studies, and possibly to major surgery, when some or all of the colon was available for direct observation. It is considered, therefore, that there would not be any appreciable increase in the number of such patients or of their intestinal tumors.

An investigation of the 83 cases with more than five adenomas showed that the group contained 58 patients whose familial and clinical histories suggested that they suffered from polyposis coli. The average number of adenomas present in the 58 patients was about 1,000, with a range of about 200 to 3,500. Among the other 25 patients with more than five adenomas, none had more than 48 tumors. In a few patients outside this particular series, counts up to 70 or 80 adenomas have been made. Similarly, there have been perhaps two cases considered to be familial polyposis with fewer than 200 adenomas but not less than 100 polyps. It would seem logical, therefore, to suggest the figure of 100 adenomas as a convenient dividing line between familial polyposis coli and what for the time being may be termed "multiple adenomas." Certainly no patient seen at St. Mark's Hospital with less than 100 adenomas has so far been found to have a relative with true familial polyposis.

This numerical difference may not be the only one between the two types of adenoma producers. Veale (1965) has postulated that all adenomas have a genetic origin. Familial polyposis coli is now known to be an inherited dominant character. Veale has suggested that the "multiple adenoma" patients, i.e., those with solitary or few adenomas, derive their tumors from the inheritance of a mendelian recessive character. This hypothesis may be an oversimplification, but it certainly goes a long way toward explaining what is known about: (1) families with an increased liability to intestinal cancer; (2) a possible mixture of early severe and late mild onset of the disease in familial polyposis patients; and (3) the relatively low incidence of intestinal cancer in colitis patients. There have been some reports of families in which there is a high incidence of intestinal cancer but no evidence of polyposis coli (Mathis, 1962; Lynch and Krush, 1967). The first systematic investigation of this problem was made by Lovett (1976), who prepared family pedigrees of patients admitted to St. Mark's Hospital with carcinoma of the colon or rectum. One-quarter of these patients had at least one other relative with intestinal cancer, and the available death certificates of deceased family members indicated an incidence of intestinal cancer four to five times greater than might be expected in the general population. Lovett also found that, where there was a strong family history of intestinal cancer, patients often had multiple adenomas, or conversely, if a patient was found to have multiple adenomas, it was not uncommon to find a high incidence of colonic and rectal cancer in the family.

The position generally appears to be that, among patients with adenomas of the large intestine, a small proportion have familial polyposis coli, which is definitely genetic in origin and associated with many hundreds of adenomas, and the great majority rarely have more than 50 adenomas and acquire these as an inherited recessive character. In this larger group it is not known how many have multiple adenomas, but study of Table 7–1 suggests that it must be at least 25 per cent. The extent to which this figure will be raised by the present policy of colonoscopy remains to be seen, but it is likely to be considerable. It might be thought trivial to be concerned with the actual number of adenomas, but experience in the last two or three decades has indicated a close relationship between adenomas and carcinomas of the large intestine—the so-called "polyp-cancer" sequence, or more accurately the "adenoma-carcinoma" sequence. One aspect of this association is the fact that, the more commonly adenomas are observed in an individual, the more probable it is that he will develop carcinoma, and the higher the risk that he will produce more than one carcinoma.

In the survey of patients with intestinal adenomas and adenocarcinomas seen at St. Mark's Hospital, patients were grouped together according to the number of adenomas present, and the incidence of carcinoma in these groups was recorded. A patient with an adenoma containing a focus of malignancy was entered under the category of "one adenoma with associated malignancy." The results are shown in Table 7–3, from which it is clear that as the number of adenomas per patient increases, so does the incidence of associated intestinal cancer in that group. It is probable that other adenomas that were present went undetected. This would have the effect of decreasing the estimated incidence of associated cancer, but it is unlikely that the relationship of this to the number of adenomas would be affected in any significant degree. The low incidence recorded in the group of 58 polyposis

TABLE 7–3 Relationship of Number of Adenomas and Incidence of Associated Carcinoma

No. of Adenomas Present	No. of Patients	No. with Associated Carcinoma	Percentage
1	1,331	395	29.7
2	296	153	51.7
3	83	47	56.6
4	40	20	50.0
5	13	10	76.9
6–48	25	20	80.0
Over 100 (Polyposis cases)	58	23	39.7
Propositus cases	31	19	61.3
Call-up cases	27	4	14.8
Total	1,846	668	36.2

TABLE 7–4 **Incidence of Multiple Synchronous and Metachronous Intestinal Cancers**

St. Mark's Hospital, 1928–1970		
Number of operation survivors	4,884	
Number with multiple synchronous cancers	197	3.2%
Number with multiple metachronous cancers	83	1.7%

patients is due to the fact that approximately half of them had been invited to attend for examination because they were known to be at risk of developing polyposis. Among the 31 propositus cases presenting because of symptoms, the incidence of cancer was 61.3 per cent.

MULTIPLE CARCINOMAS

Patients with adenomas, either the polyposis coli group or the multiple adenoma group, demonstrate the association of adenomas and carcinomas in another way—that of multiple malignant lesions. There is general agreement that, in most large series of patients with cancer of the colon or rectum, about 4 per cent will have more than one intestinal cancer. From 1928 to 1970, a total of 4,884 patients underwent excisions or resections for cancer of the colon and rectum at St. Mark's Hospital, and among these 197 (3.2 per cent) had multiple synchronous intestinal cancers (Heald and Bussey, 1975). Furthermore, 83 patients (1.7 per cent) of the original 4,884 were subsequently found to have a second intestinal cancer (Table 7–4), although it is possible that in 18 of these patients the second cancer had been present but undetected when the first cancer was located. It was noted that 75 per cent of those with multiple synchronous cancers also had adenomas; the corresponding figure for patients with metachronous cancers was 60 per cent (Heald and Lockhart-Mummery, 1972). It has to be remembered that the gross over-all figure of 1.7 per cent with metachronous carcinoma underestimates the true value, since about one-half of the group originally undergoing operations for colonic and rectal cancer probably succumbed from recurrent growth before further carcinomas could develop. If this is taken into account, the risk of a patient already operated on for an intestinal cancer developing a second growth rises to about 3.5 per cent (Bussey et al., 1967).

The association of adenomas and multiple cancers of the colon and rectum can also be shown by further analysis of the observations made on the series of St. Mark's Hospital patients seen between 1957 and 1968, the results being given in Table 7–5. It will be seen that there is a general trend for the incidence of multiple cancers to rise as the numbers of adenomas increases. Whereas in patients in whom there was

TABLE 7–5 Relationship of Number of Adenomas and Incidence of Multiple Intestinal Cancers

No. of Adenomas Present	No. of Patients	No. with Multiple Cancers	Percentage
1	1,331	25	1.9
2	296	18	6.1
3	83	12	14.5
4	40	1	2.5
5	13	3	23.1
6–48	25	8	32.0
Over 100 (Polyposis cases)	58	13	22.4
Propositus cases	31	11	35.5
Call-up cases	27	2	7.4
Total	1,846	80	4.3

evidence of only one adenoma being present, the incidence of multiple cancer was less than 2 per cent, the figure for those with more than five adenomas rises to over 30 per cent.

From what has been said so far it will not be surprising to find that multiple cancers are more common among polyposis patients than nonpolyposis patients. In a series of 151 polyposis patients with associated intestinal cancer who underwent major surgery, no less than 67 (40.8 per cent) had more than one cancer, the largest number of cancers being seven. Eleven patients in this group whose first operation removed only one carcinoma subsequently developed a further cancer in the residual large intestine, making a total of 78 patients with multiple cancers (47.6 per cent) (Bussey, 1975).

Relationship of Adenomas and Carcinomas

The frequency with which adenomas and carcinomas are found associated together indicates a close relationship. The nature of this relationship is suggested by a consideration of the frequency with which malignancy is found to arise in adenomas in three groups of cases. It has been shown that there is evidence of a benign origin in 14.2 per cent of cancers occurring singly in nonpolyposis patients (Morson, 1974). If, however, multiple cancers from nonpolyposis patients are examined in the same way, the proportion in which adenomatous tissue can be found at the periphery of the cancer rises to 27.0 per cent (Heald and Bussey, 1975). Bussey (1975) found that the cancers of the colon and rectum associated with polyposis coli (most of which occur as multiple tumors) showed an even higher proportion at 36.2 per cent (Table 7–6). The probable explanation of these figures is that most patients fail to seek medical advice until they have developed increasingly severe symptoms. When more than one carcinoma is present, the malignant tumors are usually at differing stages of development, and it is the most advanced growth that produces the necessary symptoms. Examination of the specimen obtained by subsequent surgery enables the histopathology of the carcinomas to be observed at that earlier stage when the pre-existing adenoma has not been completely destroyed by the carcinoma.

The accumulating evidence points to a close relationship between adenomas and carcinomas, one that becomes stronger as the number of adenomas increases. Some of this evidence has been obtained from observation of patients with familial polyposis coli. The use of this disease as a model for the study of the growth and behavior of adenomas is invaluable. One aspect in particular may prove to be of great importance in the control of cancer of the large intestine in the general population. At present, surgery is the only effective method of treating familial polyposis coli. If the whole large intestine is removed before there is any associated cancer, no more adenomas or cancer can arise, and the patient is cured but handicapped by a permanent ileostomy. However, if the colon only is removed and the rectum conserved to provide natural bowel functioning, it is necessary to maintain a constant watch on the rectum for new adenomas that must be destroyed by diathermy. This supervision can effectively reduce the incidence of rectal cancer to a small fraction of what it would otherwise be (see Chapter 8).

CANCER PREVENTION

No histologic differences have been reported so far between adenomas arising in patients with familial polyposis coli and the solitary or isolated adenomas found in other patients. Certainly there seems to be no difference in malignant potential for each type. The incidence of cancer among adenoma-producing patients is dependent on several factors, one of which is the number of adenomas present. It has been shown in polyposis patients that destruction of the adenomas can markedly reduce the expected incidence of rectal cancer (Bussey, 1975). A similar decrease in the cancer rate in nonpolyposis cases might be

TABLE 7–6 The Adenoma-Carcinoma Sequence

Material	Total No. of Cancers	No. with Benign Origin	Percentage
Solitary carcinoma – nonpolyposis	1,961	278	14.2
Multiple synchronous carcinoma – nonpolyposis	323	87	27.0
Solitary and multiple carcinomas – polyposis	199	72	36.2

expected if the antecedent adenomas were likewise removed. The increased use of the colonoscope has extended the benefits of the sigmoidoscope to the entire large intestine. Modifications in the instrument have improved the detection of colonic tumors, and also provided the means by which many of these growths may be effectively destroyed without the need for abdominal surgery. A major remaining problem, however, is the enormous task of locating those patients who are likely to produce adenomas. The control of cancer in polyposis patients is effective because the number of persons is small, the patients are concentrated into recognizable family groups, and diagnosis by sigmoidoscopy is easy. The nonpolyposis adenoma producers are probably a thousand times more numerous, as well as having a more scattered distribution in the general population. Colonoscopy, or barium enema examination, or both, may be required to confirm or exclude the presence of intestinal adenomas that may initially appear over a wider age-range than is the case with familial polyposis. The first requirement for the limitation of the task to practical proportions is to identify those groups or persons most at risk, and here the work of Lovett (1976) could well be a helpful beginning. Certainly the members of any family with a high incidence of intestinal cancer, and the relatives of those patients who are found to have multiple adenomas, are initial candidates for investigation and follow-up at 3- to 5-year intervals. First-degree relatives of any sufferer from colonic or rectal cancer could be another, although possibly less rewarding, line of approach. Further epidemiologic studies may indicate geographic areas of greater risk. Undoubtedly much more investigation is required before the potentiality and usefulness of widespread screening of the population in respect of intestinal cancer and its prevention can be successfully tested. If, however, some degree of concentration of these high-risk groups can be achieved, colonoscopic polypectomy could well be the means of reducing cancer incidence.

References

Bussey, H.J.R.: Familial Polyposis Coli. Johns Hopkins University Press, Baltimore, 1975.

Bussey, H.J.R., Wallace, M.H., and Morson, B.C.: Metachronous carcinoma of the large intestine and intestinal polyps. Proc. R. Soc. Med. *60*:208, 1967.

Heald, R.J., and Bussey, H.J.R.: Clinical experiences at St. Mark's Hospital with multiple synchronous cancers of the colon and rectum. Dis. Colon Rectum *18*:6, 1975.

Heald, R.J., and Lockhart-Mummery, H.E.: The lesion of the second cancer of the large bowel. Br. J. Surg. *59*:16, 1972.

Lovett, E.: Family studies in cancer of the colon and rectum. Br. J. Surg. *63*:13, 1976.

Lynch, H.T., and Krush, A.J.: Heredity and carcinoma of the colon. Am. J. Gastroenterol. *53*:517, 1967.

Mathis, M.: Familial carcinoma of the colon. A family tree from the Canton of Argau. Schweiz. Med. Wochenschr. *92*:1673, 1962.

Morson, B.C.: The polyp-cancer sequence in the large bowel. Proc. R. Soc. Med. *67*:451, 1974.

Veale, A.M.O.: Intestinal Polyposis. Eugenics Laboratory Memoirs, Series 40. Cambridge University Press, London, 1965.

Chapter Eight

Polyposis Syndromes

H. J. R. Bussey

Polyposis is defined as a condition of multiple polyps, and hence the term is a measure of the number rather than of the nature of the polyps, which should be indicated by an appropriate prefix giving the histologic type. The term "polyposis coli" is usually taken to mean "familial polyposis coli" (i.e., adenomatous polyposis), in spite of the fact that it could be applied without inaccuracy to several other conditions affecting the large intestine. These have been listed in Chapter 1 and will now be discussed in more detail.

In order to distinguish between these different forms of polyposis, a number of parameters have to be considered. These include the clinical features, other associated lesions, the number and histology of the polyps, the distribution in the gastrointestinal tract, evidence of genetic origin, and the presence or absence of associated malignant disease. Of these the most important is the histopathology of the tumors, which must be ascertained whenever possible by the excision of one or more polyps. The polyposis condition can be roughly divided into the inflammatory, hamartomatous, neoplastic, and miscellaneous groups.

INFLAMMATORY POLYPOSIS

Some inflammatory conditions of the large intestine cause severe damage to the mucosal lining, often denuding large areas at the margins of which there may be partially detached strips of mucosa. Subsequent remission of the disease with healing of the ulcers leaves these as polypoid projections or inflammatory polyps. Repeated exacerbations and remissions of the process also give rise to irregular overgrowth of the epithelium. Such circumstances are likely to occur in chronic ulcerative colitis and to a lesser extent in Crohn's disease, and because of the greater incidence of these diseases in the western world it is probable that inflammatory polyposis is numerically the most frequently encountered form of polyposis to be found in this area. The polyps are variable in number and occasionally may be present in many hundreds. Histologic examination usually shows irregularly arranged normal epithelium, inflammatory infiltration, chronic granulation tissue, and fibrosis in varying proportions. In other geographic areas where schistosomiasis is endemic, the commonest form of polyposis may also be of the inflammatory type, but due to submucosal infiltration with the parasites. Large numbers of necrotic ova are usually found in the stroma of the polyps in addition to the inflammatory infiltration.

*Benign Lymphoid Polyposis**

This is another condition that is conveniently listed among the inflammatory types. Small pale tumors, which are enlarged lymphoid follicles, may be present in large numbers throughout the gastrointestinal tract, or confined to one segment such as the large intestine. They may arise as the result of response to an inflammation or as an immunologic reaction. Since lymphoid tissue is more active in youth, a polyposis condition of this nature is more likely to be found in the earlier ages and therefore may be mistaken for familial polyposis coli, particularly if it occurs in a member of a known family (Gruenberg and Mackman, 1972). A familial incidence may be present (Louw, 1968). Prominent lymphoid follicles and Peyer's patches have been observed in the terminal ileum during the operation of colectomy for polyposis coli, and mistakenly thought to be an extension of the adenomatous colonic tumors into the small intestine.

HAMARTOMATOUS POLYPOSIS

The two most important types of hamartomatous polyp are the juvenile polyp and the Peutz-Jeghers polyp, the histologic features of which have already been described (Chapter 3). Although it is well-known that the adenomatous polyp may exist singly, in small numbers, or in hundreds as in familial polyposis coli, it is not generally appreciated that juvenile and Peutz-Jeghers polyps also occur in variable numbers. It has been known for some time that children may produce solitary or few juvenile polyps, but it was not until 1964 that the condition of juvenile polyposis coli was described by McColl et al. With

---

*See also Chapter 4.

the Peutz-Jeghers syndrome the reverse is true. The combination of gastrointestinal polyps and oral pigmentation was described about half a century ago, but it is only recently that polyps with a similar histology have been shown to occur singly or in small numbers, and without associated pigmentation. The two types of hamartomatous polyposis have certain characteristics in common.

Juvenile Polyposis

This is a rare form of polyposis that may affect the whole gastrointestinal tract or, more commonly, only the large intestine. Originally reported by McColl et al. (1964) and elaborated by Veale et al. (1966), other cases have been described since (Smilow et al., 1966; Sachatello, 1970). There is an early onset in childhood, the average age of diagnosis being about six to seven years. The main symptom is hemorrhage, the patient often suffering from severe anemia, hypoproteinemia, and underdevelopment. The number of polyps present varies from a few dozen to several hundreds. In about one-third of the families investigated there is a familial incidence, but as yet there is insufficient evidence on which to describe the nature of the inheritance. About 30 per cent of the patients have other congenital defects such as heart lesions, unusual size and shape of the skull, malrotation of the bowel, Meckel's diverticulum, undescended testis, etc. These lesions are more frequent in those patients without evidence of other affected family members. The original report of Veale et al. (1966) mentioned the possibility that one case of juvenile polyposis had occurred in an adenomatous polyposis family, but this is now considered to be incorrect and it is more likely that the other affected family members probably had juvenile polyposis also. It does seem, however, that although many of the polyps in these patients have the characteristic histology of isolated juvenile polyps as found in children, others are more atypical in their morphologic and histologic appearances, and can sometimes show dysplastic changes (usually mild) in the epithelium suggestive of adenomatous hyperplasia. Hamartomatous lesions are usually assumed not to have any malignant potential. It is not unreasonable, however, to expect this potential to be as great as that of the epithelium from which the hamartoma is derived, and possibly even increased because of the greater amount of epithelium involved. Some patients with juvenile polyposis are known to have associated large intestinal cancer, but whether this incidence is more than might be expected is the subject of current research.

Peutz-Jeghers Syndrome

The Peutz-Jeghers syndrome consists of a combination of skin pigmentation and polyps of the gastrointestinal tract. The disease is usually inherited, although "solitary" cases without any family history being encountered are the result, probably, of a new mutation. The cutaneous pigmentation consists of clusters of black or dark brown freckle-like spots, 1 to 2 mm in diameter, mainly in and around the lips and on the buccal mucosa, but often also on the fingers and toes. These spots seem to appear during the first year of life and tend to fade away in middle age. The polyps, which are counted in dozens rather than hundreds, are distributed throughout the gastrointestinal tract but are most common in the small intestine. Rarely they are limited to the large intestine. Colicky abdominal pain, usually due to intussusception of the small intestine, is the commonest symptom and usually appears in the first decade of life.

The malignant potential of the Peutz-Jeghers polyp is still being argued. Originally this was thought to be very high owing to misinterpretation of the admixture of epithelium and muscle components of the hamartoma. When the hamartomatous nature of these polyps was recognized they were said to have little or no tendency to malignant change. However, authentic cases of associated malignancy of the gastrointestinal tract have been reported, and the fact that most of these are malignancies of the stomach and duodenum probably reflects the uneven distribution around the gastrointestinal tract. Dodds et al. (1972) report two cases of colonic cancer in Peutz-Jeghers patients of the same family, but in one of these colonic adenomas were also present. It would appear that colonic cancer is a rare complication of the Peutz-Jeghers syndrome. Scully (1970) has reported that about 5 per cent of females with the Peutz-Jeghers syndrome have sex cord cell tumors of the ovary.

Other Forms of Hamartomatous Polyposis

Multiple neurofibromatosis of the gastrointestinal tract is occasionally reported in association with von Recklinghausen's disease. The tumors usually occur in the small intestine, but the colon and rectum may be involved (Levy and Khatib, 1960; Ghrist, 1963). Donnelly et al. (1969) found multiple polyps in the large intestine which proved to be a mixture of neurofibromas and juvenile polyps. Lipomatous polyposis has been encountered but must be very rare (Ling et al., 1959; Swain et al., 1969).

NEOPLASTIC POLYPOSIS

The most common neoplastic lesion to be found in the gastrointestinal tract, either single or multiple, is the adenoma. This occurs mainly in the large intestine and is the tumor responsible for the best known of the polyposis syndromes—familial polyposis coli.

Familial Polyposis Coli

In this condition many hundreds of adenomas are present throughout the colon and rectum, and because of this there is a high incidence of associated intestinal cancer. It is inherited as a dominant mendelian character which is not sex-linked. The adenomatous polyps usually begin to appear in the second and third decades of life, although later development may occur. The average number of tumors in the colon and rectum is of the order of about 1,000, most patients having between 500 and 2,500, and the range being from 150 in one case up to 5,000 in another. This numerical distribution is the reason why the figure of 100 adenomas has been suggested as a convenient distinction between familial polyposis coli and the condition termed "multiple adenomas," which is discussed later (Bussey, 1975).

The most usual symptoms are first a tendency toward increasing bowel motions, which later become associated with the passage of mucus and blood. On average, the adenomas probably are present for ten years before symptoms arise. The average age of diagnosis of polyposis in propositus cases is about 35 years. Often by then the increasing severity of the symptoms is due to intestinal cancer, which is already present in two-thirds of patients presenting for the first time. As would be expected from the large number of adenomas involved, multiple synchronous carcinomas of the colon and rectum are not uncommon; in fact, nearly one-half of the polyposis patients with associated malignant disease have more than one carcinoma.

EVOLUTION OF ADENOMAS

Familial polyposis coli is a rare disease, but there can be little doubt of its value in the study of the genetic and environmental factors involved in the production of benign and malignant epithelial tumors of the colon and rectum. One obvious example of its usefulness is the way in which histologic examination of colons affected by polyposis illustrates the early stages of adenoma formation, a process that cannot be observed elsewhere. Inspection of a colectomy specimen removed for polyposis will show numerous polyps of diminishing size, which gradually become less pedunculated until they are represented by small sessile nodules on the mucosal surface (Figs. 8–1 and 8–2). These, in turn, become so tiny as to be indistinguishable from slight irregularities in the mucous membrane on naked-eye observation. Microscopic examination, however, can identify these earlier stages of adenomas until they are no more than small collections of intramucosal tubules

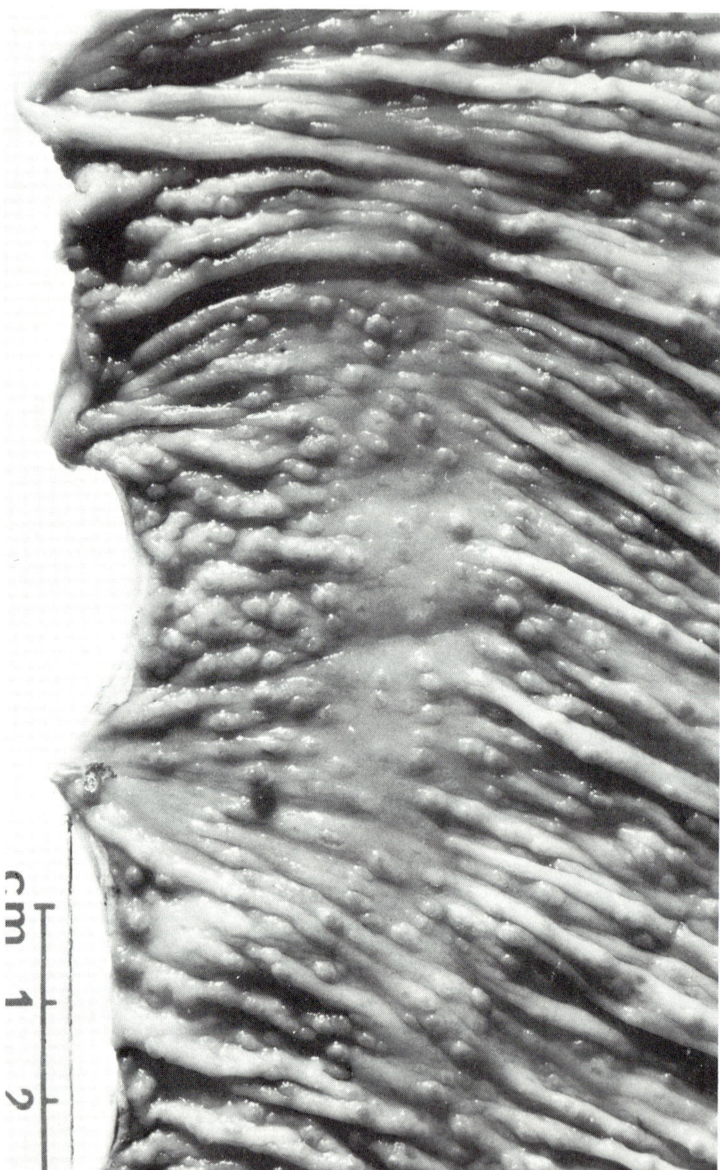

Figure 8–1 Close-up photograph of colectomy specimen removed for polyposis. Many small tumors are present, few of which are pedunculated. Most are flat mucosal nodules varying in size up to 3 mm in diameter.

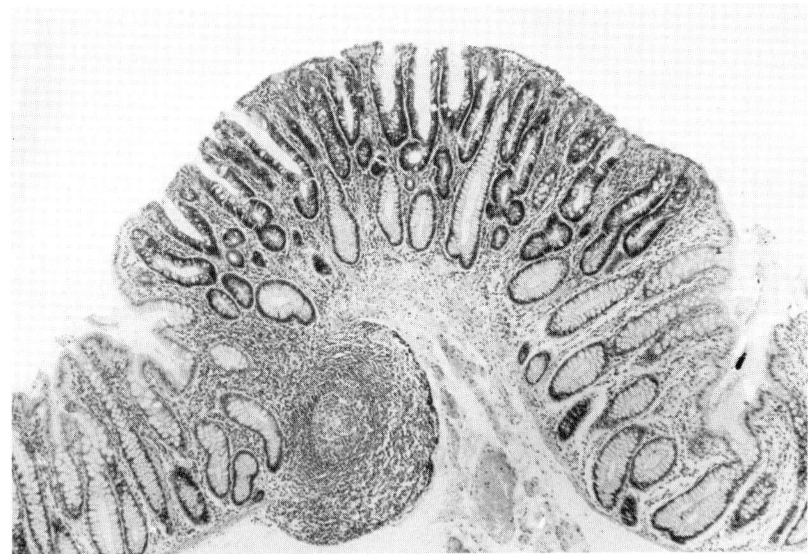

Figure 8–2 Early stage of adenoma formation. The tumor is only slightly elevated above the mucosal surface to produce a flat nodule. H&E × 70.

(Figs. 8–3 and 8–4) and, in fact, even as a single tubule (Fig. 8–5). At this point the usefulness of light microscopy in detecting the finer changes of cellular dysplasia becomes limited, and it remains to be seen if electron microscopy can be helpful in this respect. It is, however, reasonable to suggest that the steps which have been observed in the formation of adenomas in polyposis coli are also those preceding the formation of adenomas that occur either solitarily or as a few in the condition called "multiple adenomas."

THE ADENOMA-CARCINOMA SEQUENCE IN POLYPOSIS COLI

In addition to revealing the early stages in the formation of adenomatous polyps, a study of polyposis coli also adds to our information about the life history of adenomas. The age distribution at the time of diagnosis of the disease in propositus cases has been known for some time; in the St. Mark's Hospital series, the mean age is 26 to 28 years for polyposis patients without associated carcinoma, and 39.2 years when cancer is also present. For call-up members of the families found to have polyposis the respective figures are 23.7 and 33.0 years. In both groups it appears that the adenomas of polyposis exist on average for about ten years before malignancy appears. Unfortunately it is not possible to indicate the length of time before individual adenomas become malignant, but the range must be wide. There are certainly considerable differences in the growth rate of the adenomas as judged by the observation of the retained rectum in patients who have

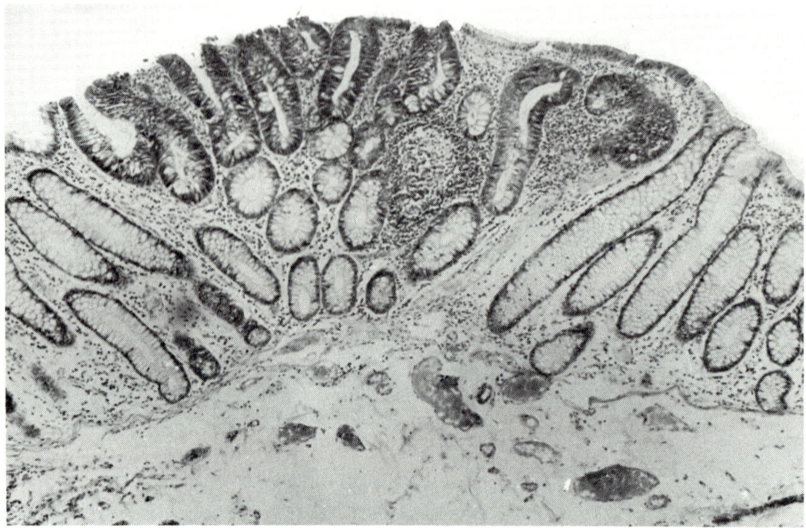

Figure 8–3 Adenomatous proliferation of the tubules is causing slight thickening of the mucosa that would not be visible to the naked eye. H&E × 70.

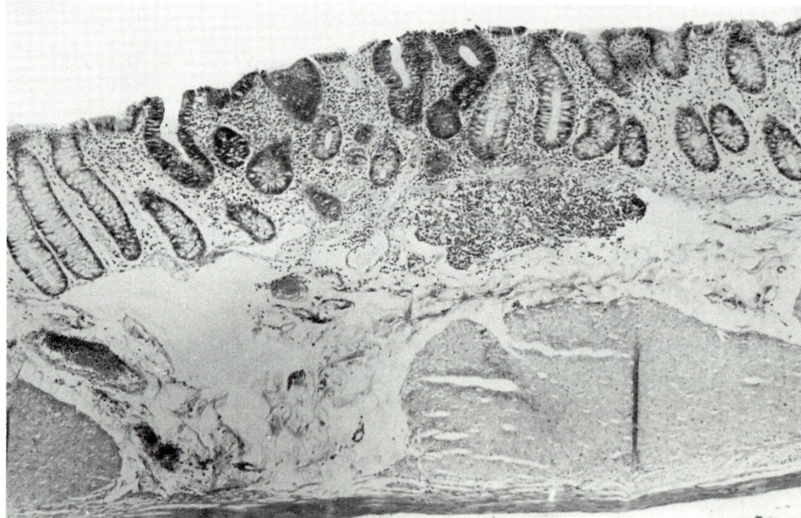

Figure 8–4 Intramucosal adenomatous changes that have not altered the thickness of the mucosa. H&E × 65.

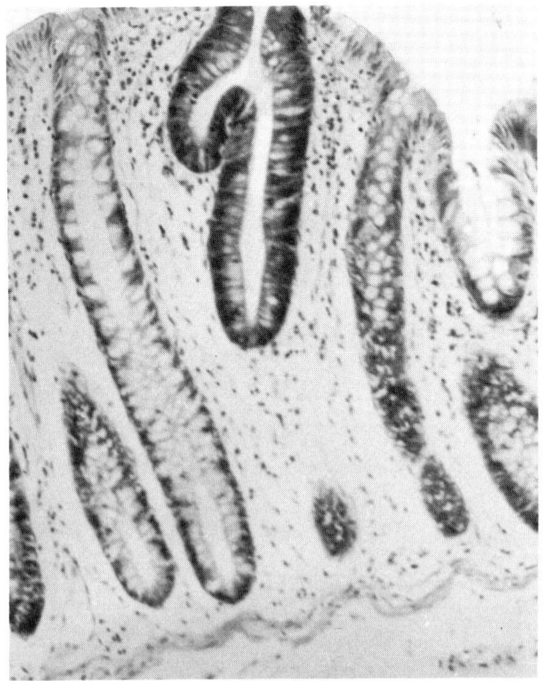

Figure 8–5 Stratification of nuclei, hyperchromatism, decreased mucus secretion, and early branching in a single crypt of Lieberkühn. H&E × 150.

undergone colectomy and ileorectal anastomosis, or in patients who have refused or postponed treatment. The increase in size of the polyps may be almost imperceptible over a period of years, or occasionally a tumor may rapidly enlarge and acquire clinical significance within a year or two. Much requires to be learned about the natural history of polyps and this information is not easily acquired.

The relationship between adenomas and cancer can also be studied in polyposis in another way. Some patients have not been treated because of their general condition or because they refused operation, and in past years some were submitted to limited surgery only. By observing when cancer appears in these patients it is possible to gain some idea of the length of the precancerous phase. There are 65 such patients in the St. Mark's Hospital Register who have been observed over varying periods of time, and the results are recorded in Table 8–1. It is clear that the longer adenomas are present in the large intestine, the more likely it is that malignancy will supervene. If the period is only five years the incidence of cancer is about 10 per cent, but around 20 years the figure is in the region of 50 per cent, and it continues to rise steadily after that time. This is in keeping with the clinical experience with the propositus cases. On the other hand, it is important to note that large

TABLE 8–1 Length of the Precancerous Phase in Familial Polyposis Coli

Period (Years)	Number of Patients Observed	Number Surviving Period Without Cancer	Number Developing Cancer in Period	Percentage Developing Cancer
0–5	65	59	6	9.2
5–10	45	35	10	22.2
10–15	23	16	7	30.4
15–20	12	8	4	33.3
20–25	7	4	3	42.6
25–30	3	1	2	66.6
30–35	1	–	1	100.0

numbers of adenomas can be present for a considerable time without cancer appearing, confirming that in general there is a long precancerous phase during which the lesions remain benign and during which cancer prevention measures may be applied.

CANCER PREVENTION

Cancer prevention in polyposis coli is dependent on treating the adenomas before these have undergone malignant change. This in turn is dependent on diagnosing the disease at the earliest time. This is helped by finding those persons at risk and constructing a family pedigree of any patient with polyposis. All siblings of the propositus are suspect and should be examined as soon as possible. It is usually easy to identify which parent has passed on the defective gene, and his or her siblings should be examined. All children of any parent with polyposis have a 50/50 chance of inheriting the disease. It is usual to begin sigmoidoscopic examinations at about the age of 14 years and, if these are negative, to repeat the examinations at two-year intervals. This policy of intercepting the progress of the disease at the earliest possible age has had the effect of reducing the initial incidence of intestinal cancer from 66 per cent in propositus cases to 7.5 per cent in the group of polyposis patients called up for examination because they were known to be at risk.

Another demonstration of cancer prevention can be seen in the method of treatment. Polyposis may be treated by total proctocolectomy and ileostomy when all risk of future intestinal cancer is removed once and for all, but at the cost to the patient of a permanent ileostomy. Alternatively, total colectomy and ileorectal anastomosis allows normal function of the bowel but with a risk of further adenomas and possibly carcinomas appearing in the retained rectum. This risk is minimized by periodic examinations of the rectum, usually every six months, and the destruction of any adenomas by excision or diathermy.

The St. Mark's Hospital records include 107 patients treated by colectomy and ileorectal anastomosis, of whom four subsequently developed rectal cancer. Analysis by an actuarial method estimates the accumulative risk of rectal cancer over a period of 25 years following colectomy to be 6.5 per cent. It is possible that this figure will be reduced in the future, but even now it compares favorably with that of the 50 per cent incidence rate to be expected in the untreated patient. This reduction, it is important to note, has been achieved by the removal of adenomas, providing further evidence of the essential part played by adenomas in the cancer sequence, and indicating a means of prevention of intestinal cancer in the general population.

Familial polyposis coli is clearly an important model for the study of the relationship of adenomas and adenocarcinoma of the large intestine. It provides an opportunity to observe the early stages in the formation of adenomas, the adenoma-adenocarcinoma sequence, and the length of the precancerous phase, and to suggest a possible form of control of intestinal cancer.

The subject of familial polyposis coli cannot be left without a reference to Gardner's syndrome. In the early 1950s Gardner and his co-workers reported a syndrome consisting of adenomatous polyposis coli, multiple osteomas of the skull and mandible, and multiple epidermoid cysts and soft tissue tumors of the skin (Gardner, 1951; Gardner and Richards, 1953). The syndrome has been modified since, both by Gardner himself (1962 and 1969) and by other workers, the principal alterations being extension of the osteomas to the whole skeleton and the addition of: (1) desmoid tumors of the abdominal wall and abdominal cavity (Smith, 1959; McAdam and Goligher, 1970); (2) diffuse fibrosis of the mesentery (Simpson et al., 1964); (3) dental abnormalities (Gardner, 1969); (4) carcinoma of the periampullary region of the duodenum (MacDonald et al., 1967; Bussey, 1972); (5) carcinoma of the thyroid (Crail, 1949; Camiel et al., 1968); and (6) malignant lesions of the central nervous system (Turcot et al., 1959). There appears to be no difference in the type of adenomatous polyposis of the colon and rectum in patients with and without the other lesions of Gardner's syndrome, and controversy continues as to whether all these associated lesions are due to the effect of one gene or involve more than one mutation. Some families show a much less clear-cut picture of Gardner's syndrome than others, and the work of Utsunomiya and Nakamura (1975) on subclinical osteomas of the mandible tends to blur the distinction further. On the other hand, some families in the St. Mark's Hospital Polyposis Register have definite adenomatous polyposis without the slightest suggestion of any of the Gardner's syndrome lesions. It may be that the latest investigations into the incidence rate of tetraploidy among fibroblasts in the skin of Gardner-type polyposis patients (Danes, 1975) and of tissue types as a marker for polyposis patients (Vargish et al., 1975) will help in the understanding of these differences.

Multiple Adenomas

It will be shown in Chapter 12 that there exists a group of patients who have adenomas, that at least one-quarter of these have more than one adenoma, and that this proportion, if polyposis is defined as a condition of having polyps, will probably qualify as patients with "adenomatous polyposis." These have already been excluded from the familial polyposis coli group on a numerical basis. It is, however, possible to make a further distinction on genetic grounds, because Veale (1965) has suggested that patients with the lesser number of intestinal adenomas may acquire them as the result of a recessive-type inheritance. The possibility of this hypothesis being true makes it difficult to suggest a scientific name that differentiates this lesion from familial polyposis coli without being too cumbersome. Since it is important to make this distinction, until the true nature of its origin is known, it has become customary to refer to the term "multiple adenomas." There is no difficulty in separating most patients in this group from the true polyposis patients, but when the adenomas are as many as 20 or 30 or more there is a tendency to diagnose the condition as familial polyposis coli, particularly as there may be an increased incidence of intestinal cancer among the relatives of such patients.

Other Types of Neoplastic Polyposis

Neoplastic lesions of the large intestine, apart from adenomas, are uncommon, and it is not surprising, therefore, that other types of polyposis due to neoplasms are rare. Multiple lymphosarcomatous polyps have been reported (Cornes, 1961; Poutasse, 1963), and in at least one patient with chronic lymphatic leukemia the initial presentation was of intestinal symptoms due to multiple polyps of the colon and rectum.

MISCELLANEOUS TYPES OF POLYPOSIS

Hyperplastic (Metaplastic) Polyposis

The hyperplastic polyp has already been described in Chapter 2. This lesion is frequently present in small numbers, but it is not generally known that the tumors may sometimes be both larger and more numerous than usual. In these circumstances a clinical diagnosis of adenomatosis may be made which will be corrected only by biopsy of the polyps, once again emphasizing the necessity of obtaining histologic confirmation of the nature of the polyps in any polyposis condition. At least ten patients with multiple hyperplastic polyps of the colon and rectum have been seen at St. Mark's Hospital to whom, at some stage of their previous clinical investigation, a label of adenomatous polyposis had been attached. As far as is known hyperplastic polyposis has no pathologic significance, is not a precancerous lesion, and has not been observed to have a familial distribution.

Cronkhite-Canada Syndrome

First described by Cronkhite and Canada (1955), little is known about this unusual condition although the number of recorded cases is increasing. It would appear to result from a metabolic disorder. The main symptoms are alopecia and nail dystrophy, accompanied by diarrhea and increase in fecal fat content. It has a grave prognosis. A condition of multiple "polyps" may be found throughout the entire gastrointestinal tract owing to cystic dilatation of the mucosal crypts, probably aggravated by edema and secondary inflammation. The condition has been mistaken for ulcerative colitis with associated colitis polyposa.

Pneumatosis Cystoides Intestinalis

Patients with this condition present with multiple cysts of the large intestine. The cysts, which are filled with gas, are situated in the submucosa and bulge the overlying mucosa into the lumen of the bowel. The radiographic appearances may resemble those of polyposis, but again biopsy and histologic examination will indicate the true diagnosis. Both in this condition and in the Cronkhite-Canada syndrome, the intestinal lesions are polypoid rather than true polyps, and appear to be secondary to more general systemic conditions.

References

Bussey, H. J. R.: Extracolonic lesions associated with polyposis coli. Proc. R. Soc. Med. *65*:294, 1972.

Bussey, H. J. R.: Familial Polyposis Coli. Johns Hopkins University Press, Baltimore, 1975.

Camiel, M. R., Mulé, J. E., Alexander, L. L., and Benninghoff, D. L.: Association of thyroid carcinoma with Gardner's syndrome in siblings. N. Engl. J. Med. *278*:1058, 1968.

Cornes, J. S.: Multiple lymphomatous polyposis of the gastrointestinal tract. Cancer *14*:249, 1961.

Crail, H. W.: Multiple primary malignancies arising in rectum, brain and thyroid. U.S. Navy Med. Bull. *49*:123, 1949.

Cronkhite, L. W., and Canada, W. J.: Generalized gastro-intestinal polyposis. Unusual syndrome of polyposis, pigmentation, alopecia and onychotrophia. N. Engl. J. Med. *252*:1011, 1955.

Danes, B. S.: The Gardner syndrome: a study in cell culture. Cancer *36*:2327, 1975.

Dodds, W. J., Schulte, W. J., Hensley, G. T., and Hogan, W. J.: Peutz-Jeghers syndrome and gastrointestinal malignancy. Am. J. Roentgenol. *115*:374, 1972.
Donnelly, W. H., Sieber, W. K., and Yunis, E. J.: Polypoid ganglioneurofibromatosis of the large bowel. Arch. Pathol. *87*:537, 1969.
Gardner, E. J.: A genetic and clinical study of intestinal polyposis, a predisposing factor for carcinoma of the colon and rectum. Am. J. Hum. Genet. *3*:167, 1951.
Gardner, E. J.: Follow-up study of a family group exhibiting dominant inheritance for a syndrome including intestinal polyps, osteomas, fibromas and epidermal cysts. Am. J. Hum. Genet. *14*:376, 1962.
Gardner, E. J.: Gardner's syndrome re-evaluated after twenty years. Proc. Utah Acad. *46*:1, 1969.
Gardner, E. J., and Richards, R. C.: Multiple cutaneous and subcutaneous lesions occurring simultaneously with hereditary polyposis and osteomatosis. Am. J. Hum. Genet. *5*:139, 1953.
Ghrist, T. D.: Gastrointestinal involvement in neurofibromatosis. Arch. Intern. Med. *112*:357, 1963.
Gruenberg, J., and Mackman, S.: Multiple lymphoid polyps in familial polyposis. Ann. Surg. *175*:552, 1972.
Levy, D., and Khatib, R.: Intestinal neurofibromatosis with malignant degeneration: a report of a case. Dis. Colon Rectum *3*:140, 1960.
Ling, C. S., Leagus, C., and St. Ahlgren, L. H.: Intestinal lipomatosis. Surgery *46*:1054, 1959.
Louw, J. H.: Polypoid lesions of the large bowel in children with particular reference to benign lymphoid polyposis. Pediatr. Surg. *3*:195, 1968.
MacDonald, J. M., Davis, W. C., Cragg, H. R., and Berk, A. D.: Gardner's syndrome and peri-ampullary malignancy. Am. J. Surg. *113*:425, 1967.
McAdam, W. A. F., and Goligher, J. C.: The occurrence of desmoids in patients with familial polyposis coli. Br. J. Surg. *57*:618, 1970.
McColl, I., Bussey, H. J. R., Veale, A. M. O., and Morson, B. C.: Juvenile polyposis coli. Proc. R. Soc. Med. *57*:896, 1964.
Moertel, C. G., Hill, J. R., and Adson, M. A.: Surgical management of multiple polyposis. Arch. Surg. *100*:521, 1970.
Poutasse, J. D.: Unusual colon manifestations of lymphosarcoma. Am. J. Dig. Dis. *8*:545, 1963.
Sachatello, C. R., Pickren, J. W., and Grace, J. T., Jr.: Generalized juvenile gastrointestinal polyposis. Gastroenterology *58*:699, 1970.
Scully, R. E.: Sex-cord tumor with annular tubules: a distinctive ovarian tumor of the Peutz-Jeghers syndrome. Cancer *25*:1107, 1970.
Simpson, R. D., Harrison, E. G., and Mayo, C. W.: Mesenteric fibromatosis in familial polyposis: a variant of Gardner's syndrome. Cancer *17*:526, 1964.
Smilow, P. C., Pryor, C. A., Jr., and Swinton, N. W.: Juvenile polyposis coli: a report of three patients in three generations of one family. Dis. Colon Rectum *9*:248, 1966.
Smith, W. G.: Desmoid tumours in familial multiple polyposis. Mayo Clin. Proc. *34*:31, 1959.
Swain, V. A. J., Young, W. F., and Pringle, E. M.: Hypertrophy of the appendices epiploicae and lipomatous polyposis of the colon. Gut *10*:587, 1969.
Turcot, J., Despres, J. P., and St. Pierre, F.: Malignant tumors of the central nervous system associated with familial polyposis of the colon. Dis. Colon Rectum *2*:465, 1959.
Utsunomiya, J., and Nakamura, T.: The occult osteomatous changes in the mandible in patients with familial polyposis coli. Br. J. Surg. *62*:45, 1975.
Vargish, T., Dawkins, H. G., Jr., Heise, E., and Myers, R. T.: Serologic detection of persons at risk in familial polyposis coli. Surg. Forum, Vol. XXVI, 61st Annual Clinical Congress 1975, Am. Coll. Surg.
Veale, A. M. O.: International Polyposis. Eugenics Laboratory Memoirs, Series 40. Cambridge University Press, London, 1965.
Veale, A. M. O.: Intestinal Polyposis. Eugenics Laboratory Memoirs. Series 40. Cambridge University Press, London, 1965.
Veale, A. M. O., McColl, I., Bussey, H. J. R., and Morson, B. C.: Juvenile polyposis coli. J. Med. Genet. *3*:5, 1966.

Chapter Nine

Precancer in Ulcerative Colitis

R. H. Riddell, D. C. Shove, J. K. Ritchie, J. E. Lennard-Jones, and B. C. Morson

Carcinoma that complicates ulcerative colitis accounts for only a very small proportion of all large bowel carcinomas; the true figure is probably less than 1 per cent. It has been estimated that there were approximately 100,000 new cases of large bowel cancer in the U.S.A. in 1975 (American Cancer Society, 1974). Based on this figure only about 1,000 arose as a complication of ulcerative colitis. It could reasonably be asked then why such a disproportionate amount of interest should be shown in these few cases. The answer is not difficult to find, for these patients, although few in number, pose a real problem in management. The main reasons for this are that the carcinomas develop insidiously even when patients are under active medical care, are frequently multiple, and may not become clinically apparent until the lesion is well advanced, when only palliation can be offered. Diagnosis is difficult because many of these cancers are flat or plaque-like and this makes them difficult to recognize either radiologically or endoscopically. The average age at which they are discovered is 40 to 45, which is earlier than noncolitic cancers, although the average age at death (46) may be a more accurate index (Mottet, 1971). There is a group of patients with total or extensive colitis, an early age of onset, and a long history of symptoms among whom virtually all of the cancers occur.

Total disease requires no elaboration, and extensive disease is defined as involvement to the hepatic flexure as demonstrated radiologically. This immediately raises the question whether radiologic examination is a reliable indicator of the extent of disease. Dilaware et al. (1973) have shown that endoscopy and biopsy are invariably superior to radiologic examination in determining the extent of colitis. Carcinoma occurring in patients with distal colitis only is very rare, and probably of similar incidence to that arising in the noncolitic population (Hinton, 1966).

It is commonly stated that carcinoma rarely arises in patients with colitis before the disease has been present for ten years. This assumes that the date of onset of symptoms can always be recorded accurately. Mottet (1971), by combining several series, has shown that 22 per cent of all cases develop with a history of less than ten years. However, the direct relationship between the length of history and the incidence of carcinoma is not in doubt (Edwards and Truelove, 1964; Goligher et al., 1968), and the figure of ten years is now generally accepted.

There is evidence that patients whose disease begins before the age of 25 are at increased risk of developing carcinoma (MacDougall, 1964a, b), and that the highest risk is with onset of symptoms in childhood (Devroede et al., 1973). In one series, 17 per cent of children with ulcerative colitis went on to develop carcinoma (Rosenqvist et al., 1959).

Other factors that have been suggested as predisposing to cancer are a severe first attack (Edwards and Truelove, 1964) and the character of the symptomatology. These authors consider that chronic, continuous symptoms predispose to carcinoma; Svartz and Ernberg (1949) suggested that patients with long-standing quiescent colitis are at greatest risk. Goligher (1968) has encountered both situations.

Yeomans, as early as 1927, when describing only the second case of carcinoma developing in ulcerative colitis (the first having been described two years before by Crohn and Rosenburg), raised the possibility that carcinoma might be related to the development of inflammatory polyps. This view, now regarded as erroneous, was expounded by numerous authors subsequently, and the entire sequence and previous literature were well described by Dawson and Pryse-Davies (1959).

In 1967, Morson and Pang described "precancerous" epithelial changes in rectal biopsies from patients with a long history of colitis. Examination of colectomy specimens showed that this epithelial atypia or dysplasia was often extensive, and involved the mucosa away from the site of the carcinoma as well as in its immediate vicinity. Similar changes were found in a retrospective study of 12 of 134 patients with pancolitis undergoing subsequent resection, an incidence of 9 per cent. In nine patients a report of premalignant change in the preoperative rectal biopsy was responsible to some extent for subsequent proctocolectomy, and in five of these an occult carcinoma was found in the resection specimen. This supported the theory of a detectable preinvasive phase and suggested that, because the changes were widespread and mostly involved the distal bowel, rectal biopsy might be of value in determining which patients within the clinical high-risk group of colitics were most likely to develop cancer; indeed, it is apparent that when precancerous changes were present there was already something like a 50 per cent chance that a small carcinoma had already developed. The predominance of Dukes stage A cases among them suggested that well over 95 per cent of these patients could be cured of their disease. This work was confirmed by Hulten et al. (1972) and Myrvold et al. (1974), who described 47 patients with ulcerative colitis treated by proctocolectomy from whom rectal biopsies had been taken prior to operation. In seven of these premalignant change was found in the rectal biopsies, and when the subsequent resection specimen was examined a carcinoma was found in five, whereas it had only been suspected clinically in one. Evans and Pollock (1972) pointed out that cancer could develop in long-standing colitis in the absence of precancerous epithelial dysplasia, and that rectal biopsy might not always be helpful.

DISTRIBUTION OF CARCINOMAS IN ULCERATIVE COLITIS

The site and sex of colitic cancers are shown in Table 9–1. It is noteworthy that the rectum is by far the most common site, and that proportionately this was more marked in males (47.8 per cent) than in females (39.9 per cent). This is in keeping with, although somewhat less than, carcinomas occurring in noncolitic patients, in whom over-all most cancers occur in the rectum in males and more commonly affect the colon in females. When patients whose cancers occurred singly are separated from those with multiple tumors (Table 9–2), and the distributions compared, it is apparent that there is little difference between the sexes in the distribution of multiple tumors; however, when single cancers are considered there is a marked predominance of rectal cancers in men, whereas women show a much greater tendency to develop tumors proximal to the rectum. The pattern of multiple tumors was examined to see if there was any particular distributional tendency,

TABLE 9–1 Site and Sex of 111 Carcinomas Arising in Ulcerative Colitis

	Male (30 Patients)	Female (43 Patients)	Total	% of Total
Cecum	4	2	6	5.4
Ascending colon	2	1	3	2.7
Hepatic flexure	0	5	5	4.5
Transverse colon	6	13	19	17.1
Splenic flexure	3	7	10	9.0
Descending colon	6	6	12	10.8
Sigmoid colon	3	7	10	9.0
Rectum	22	24	46	41.5
Total	46	65	111	100.0

TABLE 9–2 Comparison Between Males and Females of the Distribution of Single and Multiple Tumors

	Multiple Tumors		Single Tumors	
	Male (8 Patients)	*Female (9 Patients)*	*Male (21 Patients)*	*Female (34 Patients)*
Cecum	3	1	1	1
Ascending colon	1	0	1	1
Hepatic flexure	0	4	0	1
Transverse colon	6	6	0	7
Splenic flexure	2	4	1	3
Descending colon	5	2	1	4
Sigmoid colon	2	6	1	1
Rectum	6	8	16	16
Total	25	31	21	34

but this appeared to be entirely random. It is of interest that, among the 18 patients with multiple tumors (24.7 per cent of the entire group), there were eight double tumors, five triple tumors, two patients with four tumors, one with five, and one with eight.

From these data, which are very similar to those obtained by Mottet (1971) when he combined several series, the nature of the problem of colitic cancers becomes a little clearer, for 40 per cent of the carcinomas that develop will be within reach of the sigmoidoscope, and potentially detectable by rectal biopsy. It is in the remaining 60 per cent that the presence of rectal dysplasia might be a warning of present or impending proximal malignancy.

HISTOLOGY OF PRECANCER IN COLITIS

There are five main patterns of epithelial atypia (dysplasia), two of which, adenomatous change and basal cell change, are the most common. Those that are here called in situ anaplasia, clear cell change, and pancellular change are relatively infrequent (Riddell, 1976).

Adenomatous Change

This is the usual histologic picture of dysplasia in colitis (Fig. 2). It is found in mucosa of either normal or increased thickness; it may be diffuse or patchy, and gives a macroscopic appearance of small, warty excrescences or a nodular and velvety surface (Fig. 9–1), in which the full spectrum of adenomatous change from villous through tubulovillous to tubular adenoma may be seen. Exceptionally, a localized or

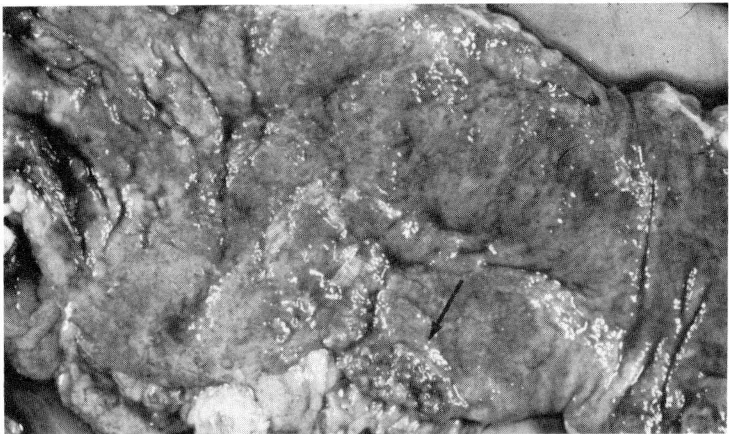

Figure 9–1 Early carcinoma in ulcerative colitis: note the nodular area (*arrow*) in the sigmoid colon beneath which there was a colloid carcinoma. Although this appearance is virtually never seen in noncolitics, it is relatively common in the colitic population.

polypoid form may be indistinguishable from an adenoma arising in noncolitic mucosa.

When a villous mucosa is present there is little branching of crypts, and the villi vary from short and stubby to long and slender (Fig. 9–2). There is some relationship between villous height and the degree of dysplasia, for severe dysplasia is uncommon in long, slender villi. Furthermore, long villi often show evidence of maturation as the luminal surface is approached, so that the most severe dysplasia is seen in the crypts. As the villi become shorter and eventually disappear, the dysplastic crypts become more readily bifid and budding may also be present (Fig. 9–3). This can be sufficiently marked to produce a "back-to-back" appearance of adjacent glands. A further feature best appreciated at low power is the amount of mucus present in the epithelium. This bears a close relationship to the degree of dysplasia, which is hardly surprising, for the production of goblet cells must reflect to some extent the ability of the mucosa to undergo maturation, and this is least well seen in the most dysplastic mucosa. Under these circumstances, the cytoplasm may be uniformly eosinophilic (Fig. 9–2*B*). When there is mild dysplasia, more goblet cells are apparent, and these are usually individual. However, on occasion this may take the form of a row of cells in which the mucus droplet occupies only the luminal border.

Cytologically, cell size is uniform and the nuclei show all the usual features of dysplasia, being elongated, hyperchromatic, pleomorphic, and overlapping, with loss of polarity so that they come to occupy a more luminal position in the cell (Fig. 9–2*B*). Small nucleoli may occasionally be seen. Sometimes the nuclei are more open and vesicular, with a dense, peripheral chromatin ring and one or two eosinophilic nucleoli

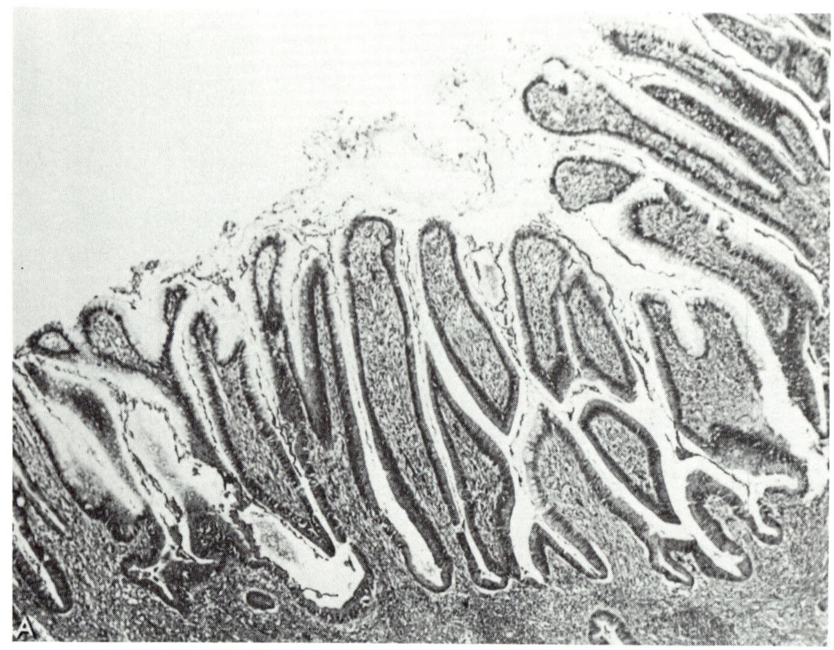

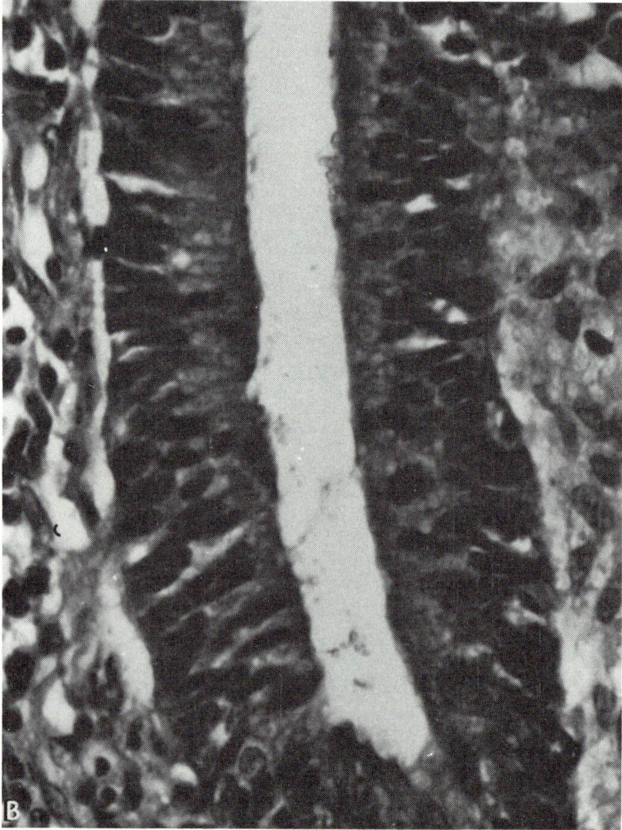

Figure 9–2 *See legend on opposite page.*

that can be very prominent (Fig. 9–4). Mitotic figures are sometimes numerous but on other occasions are very difficult to find. Mitoses in the mouths of crypts are very rare in non-neoplastic mucosa unless these are also accompanying surface ulceration. Paneth and argentaffin cells are infrequent in this type of dysplasia, and where this is focal the change from the typical picture of chronic ulcerative colitis with Paneth cell metaplasia to a dysplastic mucosa is usually marked by an abrupt cessation of Paneth and argentaffin cells.

*Basal Cell Change**

This is seen in mucosa of normal thickness which macroscopically, other than being flat and atrophic, is relatively featureless; thus, there is no indication of its presence on gross inspection and the diagnosis is histologic. Rarely, a similar change may be found in villous mucosa. Sometimes it is found admixed with the adenomatous type of dysplasia in areas of severe dysplasia. Microscopically, cell size is normal or only slightly increased, but the characteristic feature of this type of change is the presence of a row of small prominent nuclei with moderate or marked hyperchromatism. Pleomorphism is minimal and there is no tendency to stratification. The nuclei do not assume a more luminal position or lose their polarity and remain basal in position. The low-power appearance is, therefore, distinct and unusual, and resembles Beluga caviar arranged in a row (Fig. 9–4). Under high power or oil immersion many of the nuclei can be seen to have a dense peripheral chromatin rim, a prominent nucleolus, and polychromatism, with variation in hyperchromicity between nuclei. The cytoplasm is similarly distinct and is markedly eosinophilic, largely owing to the virtual absence of goblet cells, which again probably reflects the inability of these cells to undergo maturation; however, from time to time there is a suggestion of maturation as indicated by the presence of a small row of mucin droplets close to the luminal border of the cells. The impression then is that cells traverse the length of the crypt without evidence of maturation, and for this reason the appearance has been termed "basal cell change." The number of mitotic figures is very variable, but they are readily identified.

*See Figure 9–4.

Figure 9–2 *A*, Adenomatous change of villous type. The villi are tall and slender, but the greatest degree of dysplasia is often seen at the base of the crypts, with evidence of maturation as the surface is approached. H & E × 35. *B*, High power of a crypt base showing typical adenomatous features. H & E × 700.

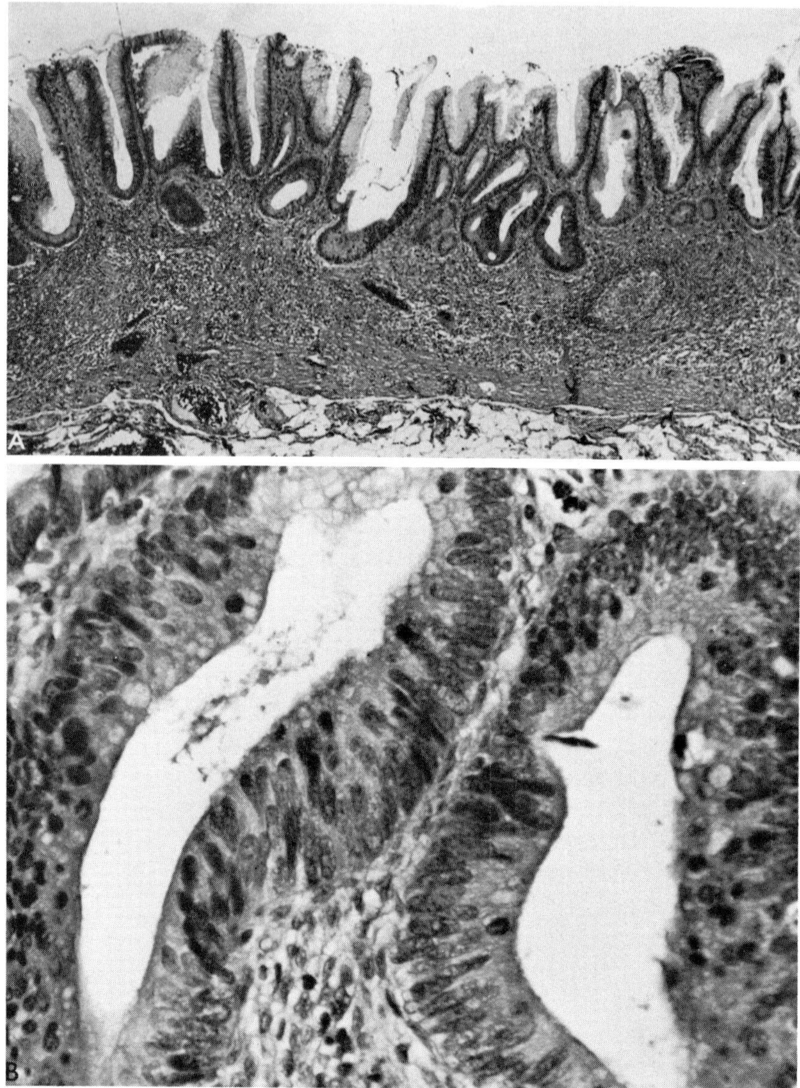

Figure 9–3 *A,* Adenomatous change of tubular type. This example is a little unusual in showing maximal dysplasia in the crypt bases as seen in the more villous mucosa, with much mucin production in the mouth of the crypts. Note the distortion and branching at the crypts base. In this type the maximum dysplasia is more usually at the surface. H & E × 75. *B,* High power of crypt bases showing typical adenomatous features. H & E × 700.

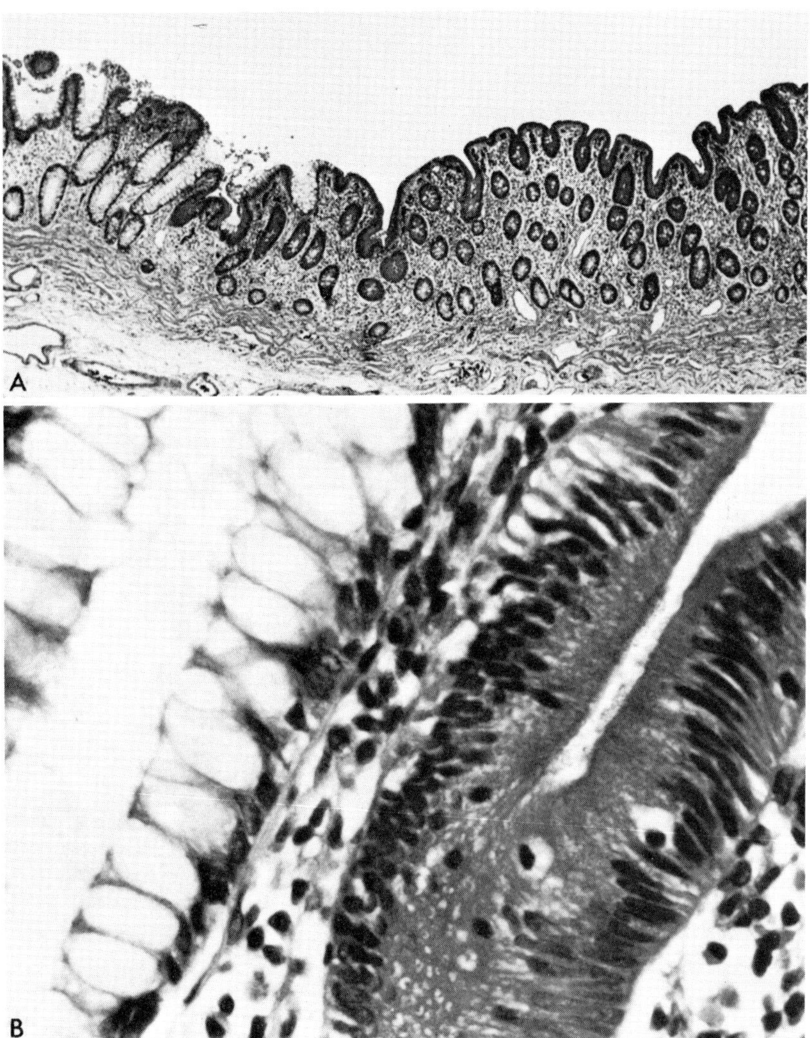

Figure 9–4 *A*, Basal cell change in low power. There is an abrupt change from typical colitic mucosa in the six crypts on the extreme left to the very eosinophilic crypts in the remainder of the section. H & E × 35. *B*, High power of the junctional region to allow comparision between the two crypt types. H & E × 700.

Argentaffin cells are not infrequent and Paneth cells may also be found, particularly when dysplasia is not severe. There usually is little increase in the inflammatory cell content of the lamina propria. It seems to be this type of mucosa that readily gives rise to so many of the poorly differentiated and signet ring cell tumors that characterize ulcerative colitis (Figs. 9–5 and 9–6). A further feature of interest is that, when this type of mucosa gives rise to a carcinoma, there is often infiltration of the lamina propria, a feature more characteristic of gastric than colonic cancer.

In Situ Anaplasia

This is rare, and when present is usually associated with the basal cell type of change described above. It is unrecognizable macroscopically, but microscopically takes one of two forms. There is either a breakdown of crypt architecture so that small foci of carcinoma are present solely in the mucosa (Fig. 9–7), or very little recognizable crypt architecture, and the mucosa is entirely replaced by numerous, small, undifferentiated or signet ring cells (Fig. 9–8).

Clear Cell Type

In contrast to in situ anaplasia, this change is open to misinterpretation because of its apparent innocence. It is characterized by large,

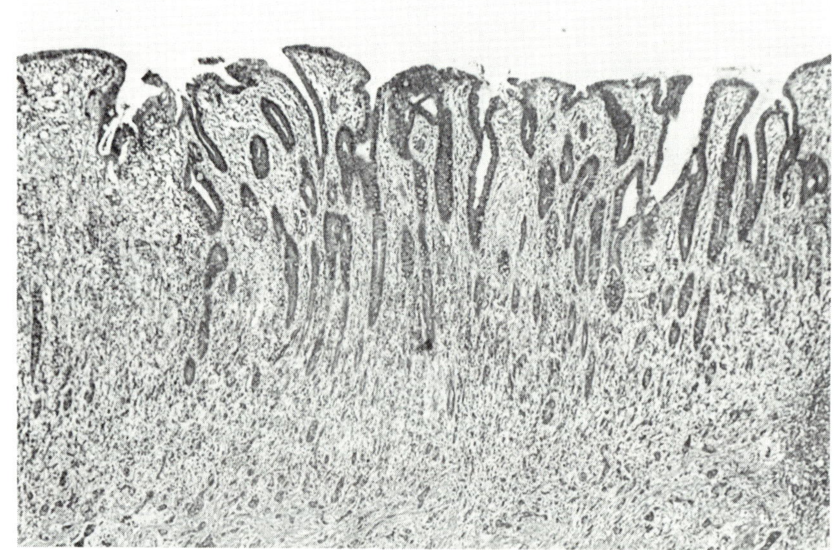

Figure 9–5 Poorly differentiated carcinoma arising from attenuated crypts. This was also a plaque and no surface ulceration was present. H & E × 30.

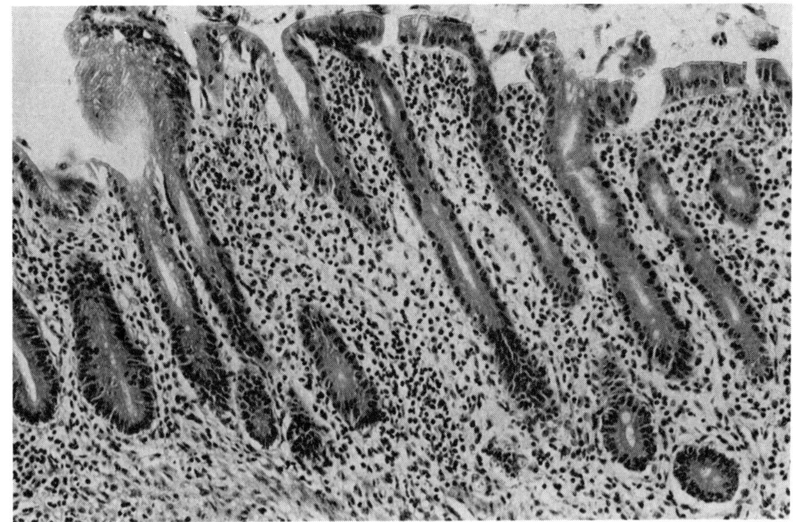

Figure 9–6 Mucosa adjacent to the carcinoma of Fig. 9–5. Note the narrow elongated crypts with a narrow lumen, and the deeply staining cytoplasm with absence of goblet cells. The characteristic nuclei are apparent even at this magnification. Note also the moderate increase in mononuclear cells in the lamina propria. H & E × 120.

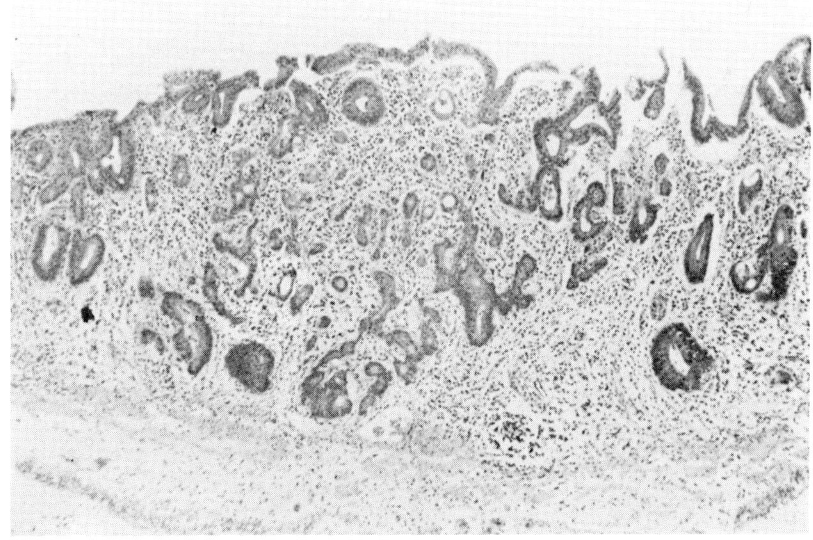

Figure 9–7 Focus of intramucosal carcinoma. H & E × 75.

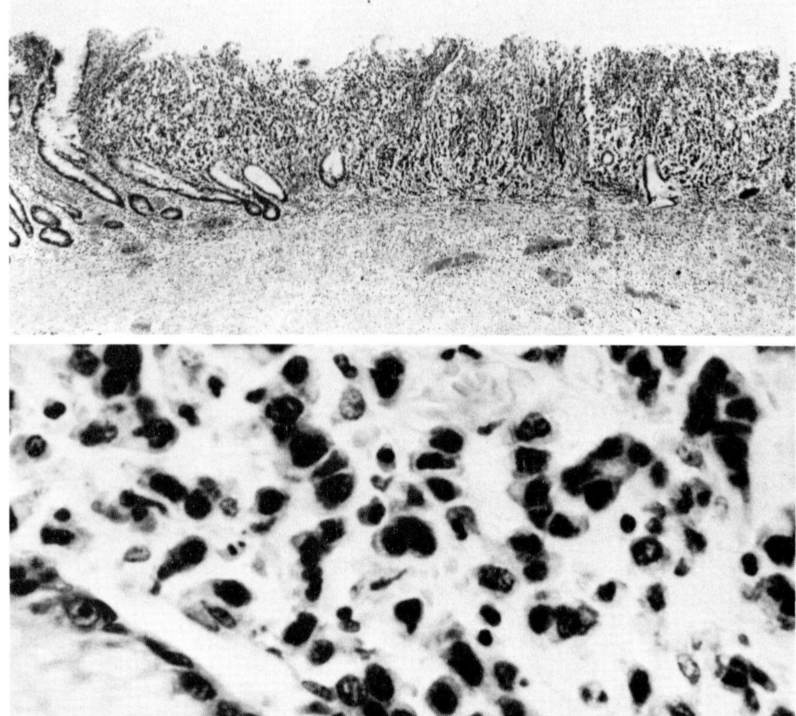

Figure 9–8 In situ anaplasia. Occasional residual crypts can be seen close to the muscularis mucosae. H & E × 30. Lower half of the figure shows a high-power view of the intramucosal undifferentiated small cell carcinoma. Part of a residual crypt is seen in the bottom left corner. H & E × 80.

clear cells, which stain poorly with either alcian blue (pH 2.5) or by the PAS diastase method. The nuclei are elongated and hyperchromatic, and there is some loss of polarity (Fig. 9–9). Carcinomas arising from this type tend to be well-differentiated (Fig. 9–10). Close to the surface the lumen takes on an irregular arrangement that is reminiscent of the sawtooth arrangement seen in hyperplastic polyps. Paneth and argentaffin cells are not seen, and mitotic figures are rare.

Pancellular Change

This is characterized by dysplasia that is manifest mainly as large hyperchromatic nuclei with loss of polarity, but this affects all cell lines, including Paneth, argentaffin, and goblet cells. Paneth cells are prominent (Fig. 9–11), are found away from their usual position at the base of the crypts, and appear to be migrating up the crypt. Argentaffin

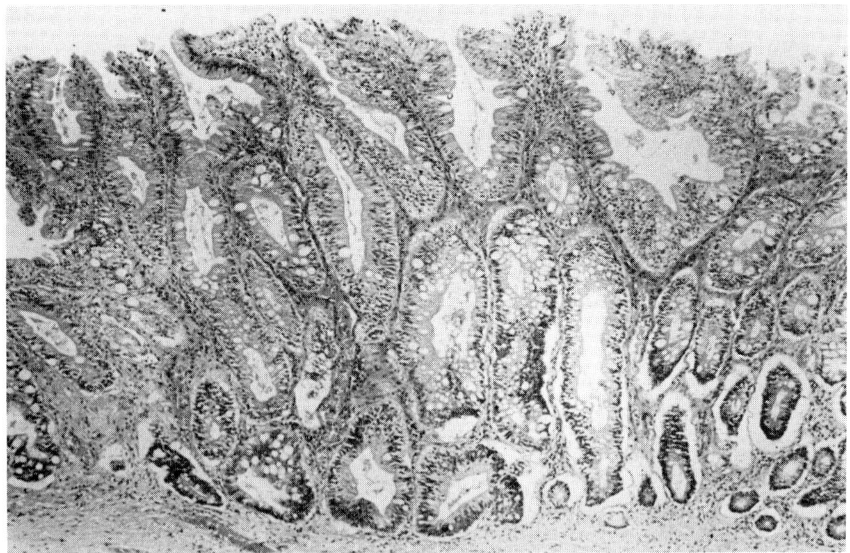

Figure 9–9 Clear cell change: part of a mucosal nodule showing large, tightly packed crypts with mild nuclear abnormality. H & E × 75.

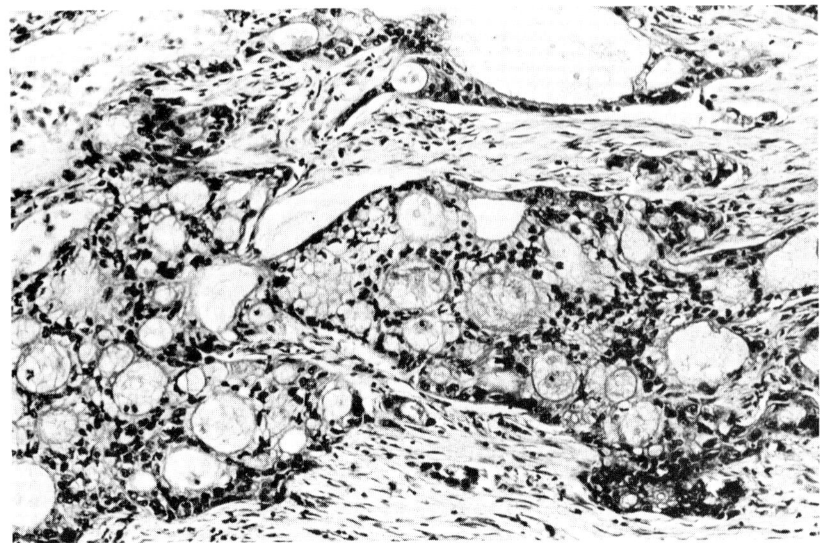

Figure 9–10 Well-differentiated goblet cell carcinoma that was in continuity with a focus of dysplasia very similar to that seen in Fig. 9–14. H & E × 120.

cells also appear far more numerous and entirely surround the crypt, giving an appearance resembling an in situ argentaffinoma. Goblet cells tend to be distended with mucus, possibly an indication of an abnormality in the normal release meachanism, and the nucleus loses its polarity and appears as a crescent at the luminal border. The comparison with a signet ring cell is unavoidable.

Finally, it should be stressed that, whereas most tumors could be seen to originate from one of these four distinctive mucosal types, this was not always so, and mixtures were often seen, particularly between the two common forms. Furthermore, when mucosa remote from the cancer was examined it was common to find different types and grades of dysplasia, although one type usually predominated.

DYSPLASIA IN THE RECTUM

If rectal biopsy is to be used to indicate which patients within the clinical high-risk group are particularly likely to develop carcinoma, it is important to know how often and to what extent the rectum becomes involved by dysplasia. It is also necessary to redefine what a positive biopsy implies. Rectal dysplasia was initially noted by Morson and Pang (1967) as a frequent and widespread change in patients with carcinoma complicating colitis which often extended to the rectum. However, it has also been shown (Table 9–1) that 40 per cent of the cancers occurring in ulcerative colitis arise in the rectum, and these should be detectable by regular sigmoidoscopy and biopsy. Furthermore, it would be expected that, if no gross lesion is seen sigmoidoscopically and random rectal biopsies are carried out at each visit, the development of these tumors could be anticipated by the finding of dysplasia. In principle, 40 per cent of the carcinomas complicating ulcerative colitis could be anticipated by these means.

The remaining 60 per cent of carcinomas developing proximal to the rectum pose a different problem: if rectal dysplasia is to be used as an indicator of proximal carcinoma, the assumption is made that the rectal changes develop at the same time as, or possibly before, the carcinoma, and it is pertinent to ask whether this is the case. If rectal biopsy is also to be used to indicate which patients have proximal dysplasia, there is an assumption that the dysplasia begins distally, and it is necessary to question whether this is so. Furthermore, it is valid to ask whether these changes are focal or diffuse, as this distinction will affect the value of rectal biopsy.

A study of the frequency and extent of rectal dysplasia was made on 63 proctocolectomy specimens removed for ulcerative colitis, and in which either a carcinoma or dysplasia was also present. The slides from the rectum were examined using an eyepiece micrometer so that the actual percentage of dysplasia could be estimated in each. In many

TABLE 9–3 Proportion of Rectal Mucosa Affected by Neoplastic Transformation in 63 Patients with Dysplasia or Carcinoma

	None	1–25%	26–50%	51–75%	76–99%	All	Total
Rectal carcinoma	0	4	7	9	4	2	26
Colon carcinoma	2	0	2	4	1	6	15
Dysplasia only	1	4	2	7	5	3	22

patients, "swiss roll" sections had been taken allowing the examination of long strips of mucosa. The results are shown in Tables 9–3 and 9–4. From these data, it is apparent that rectal dysplasia is often a patchy lesion even when a rectal carcinoma is present. When there is a proximal carcinoma or proximal dysplasia, rectal involvement with dysplasia is usually, but not invariably, present. This has several practical implications. Because dysplasia may be focal it is desirable to take multiple biopsies in order to reduce the sampling error. When multiple biopsies are being used to detect rectal dysplasia, their site should be deliberately varied at each follow-up visit to further reduce this problem. This implies that a record must be kept of the actual site of each biopsy taken. Another advantage of documenting the biopsy sites accurately is that, if only one of several taken shows dysplasia and its site of origin is known, it is easy to return to that site to take further biopsies if there is any doubt. Approximately 60 per cent of all carcinomas occurring in ulcerative colitis arise in the colon, and in the entire colitic population about 8 per cent of the expected carcinomas will occur in the absence of rectal dysplasia. Conversely, 92 per cent will show evidence of rectal dysplasia. This suggests that regular biopsies are potentially valuable, but only if the sampling error is kept to an absolute minimum by taking several biopsies and varying the biopsy sites at subsequent examinations. The only other reasonable method of detecting these changes is by colonoscopy with multiple biopsies. To submit the entire high-risk colitic group to annual or biannual colonoscopy in order to detect this small population with no rectal dysplasia may be impracticable, although several studies are currently being carried out to assess this. However, apart from detecting the small group of patients with carcinoma, but no

TABLE 9–4 Over-all Proportion of Rectal Mucosa Affected by Dysplasia and Carcinoma

	No. of Patients	Average No. of Slides	% Dysplasia	% Carcinoma
Rectal carcinoma	26	5.2	54	23
Colon carcinoma	15	2.2	69	0
Dysplasia only	22	3.1	59	0

rectal dysplasia, colonoscopy has a further advantage in that proximal dysplasia before the rectum is involved can also be detected. Excision at this stage must be contemplated, because it is possible for a small carcinoma to remain undetected colonoscopically, especially if it is a plaque-like lesion. Theoretically, and especially if the colitis has been quiescent for a long time, the question will arise as to whether dysplasia with rectal sparing can be treated by colectomy and ileorectal anastomosis. This should be discouraged, for apart from the possibility of exacerbating the colitis, the patient may develop a carcinoma in the residual rectum (Hulten et al., 1971). Should this approach be used, it is imperative that the patient be kept under very close supervision for evidence of rectal dysplasia.

GRADING DYSPLASIA IN RECTAL AND COLONIC BIOPSIES AND THE DISTINCTION FROM REACTIVE HYPERPLASIA

In normal colonic mucosa the nuclei in the crypts are very small and indistinct, and close to the basal portion of the cell. Goblet cell nuclei may sometimes be distinguished from absorptive cell nuclei by their tendency to be more hyperchromatic and shaped like an inverted flask. There is an increase in the size of the absorptive cell nuclei as the luminal surface is approached. In the acute or active phase of ulcerative colitis (Price and Morson, 1975), the nuclei are enlarged and vesicular with a light, peripheral chromatin rim, and the nucleolus becomes prominent. These features of reactive hyperplasia are seen throughout the mucosa, and particularly in epithelium undergoing active regeneration. It is apparent that the presence of large vesicular nuclei with prominent nucleoli can be a normal feature of the acute phase of ulcerative colitis, and could be confused with early or mild dysplasia.

Morson and Pang (1967) described the features of severe dysplasia that are usually present in the colon of patients with cancer complicating colitis. Subsequent studies (Hulten, Kewenter, and Ahren, 1972; Yardley and Keren, 1974; Cook and Goligher, 1975; Riddell, 1976) have further clarified the differences between mild, moderate, and severe degrees of dysplasia and the distinction from reactive hyperplasia. These are summarized in Table 9–5. Tubular or villous architecture (adenomatous change) is manifested as elongation of crypts, budding, or a villous surface configuration as previously described. Abnormalities of epithelial cells and inflammation are defined as follows:-

(a) *Nucleus.* Increase in size. Variation in size and shape.

(b) *Chromatin.* Increase in amount. Abnormality of pattern. Variation between cells.

(c) *Nucleoli.* Increase in size or number.

(d) *Mitoses.* Abnormal mitotic figures. Mitoses in upper third of crypt or on surface.

TABLE 9–5*

	Dysplasia		No Dysplasia	
	Severe (Precancer)	*Moderate or Mild*	*Reactive Hyperplasia*	*Minimal Inflammation*
TUBULAR ARCHITECTURE				
Villous change	28	14	8	0
Budding	81	15	4	0
ABNORMALITY OF EPITHELIAL CELLS				
Increased size of nucleus	100	99	100	33
Variation in size of nucleus	100	86	96	33
Variation in shape of nucleus	100	85	96	24
Increased chromatin	100	73	96	5
Abnormal chromatin	100	82	92	0
Prominent nucleoli	53	41	46	5
Increased number of nucleoli	47	29	33	0
Abnormal mitotic figures	34	0	0	0
Stratification	100	78	96	57
Increased nuclear-cytoplasmic ratio	100	95	67	14
Abnormal position of mucin	100	95	79	10
DISPOSITION OF ABNORMAL CELLS				
Mitoses in upper third of tubule	75	48	8	0
Abnormal cells in upper third of tubule	100	81	33	0
INFLAMMATION				
Acute	19	38	79	0
Chronic	72	68	100	14

*Individual criteria (percentage incidence) graded as present (1, 2, 3) or absent (0) in all 32 biopsies classified as severe dysplasia, all 73 biopsies classified as mild to moderate dysplasia, and representative samples of biopsies with no dysplasia (24 with reactive hyperplasia and 21 without).

(e) *Nucleus in relation to cytoplasm.* Variation of position within cells. Stratification of nuclei. Increase in nuclear/cytoplasmic ratio.

(f) *Goblet cells.* Mucin in some goblet cells wrongly positioned deep in the epithelial membrane instead of in its normal position along the luminal border; mucin may also lie beside the nucleus or between the nucleus and the basement membrane, rather than at the apex of the cell.

(g) *Site of abnormal cells.* Presence in upper third of tubule or on surface.

(h) *Inflammation.* Polymorphs in surface exudate, within tubules, in epithelial cell layer, and in lamina propria (active inflammation). Number of mononuclear cells in lamina propria (chronic inflammation).

Each of these criteria was graded as absent, mild, moderate, or severe according to the degree and extent of the changes within the biopsy. The differences between biopsies showing severe and moderate degrees of dysplasia, inflammatory hyperplasia, and none of these features are compared in Table 9–5. It will be seen that there is a clear difference between the characteristics of biopsies without dysplasia in the presence of minimal inflammation and those of the other three groups. However, there are many similarities between reactive hyperplasia and dysplasia of both grades. The distinction between severe and moderate dysplasia, as expected, is one of degree.

The results of the analysis of all the biopsies categorized as severe dysplasia are shown in Table 9–7.

Reference to Tables 9–6 and 9–7 shows that some abnormality of tubular architecture was present in 28 of 32 biopsies with severe dysplasia, budding being more common than villous change. Abnormal mitoses, although infrequently seen, were found only in this group. Abnormal cells were present in the upper third of the tubules in all 32 biopsies, and mitoses were seen at this site in three-quarters. From this analysis, these five criteria appear to be the most important in distinguishing severe dysplasia from both lesser degrees of dysplasia and reactive hyperplasia.

VALUE OF RECTAL AND COLONIC BIOPSY

The clinical outcome in patients with and without dysplasia on biopsy has been studied by Lennard-Jones et al., 1977. They found no carcinoma in a group of patients without dysplasia during 941 patient-years of follow-up. For patients with mild or moderate dysplasia the outcome is shown in Table 9–6. Dysplasia was found in only three patients whose length of history was less than eight years.

In 13 patients, severe dysplasia was recognized in one or more biopsies. The outcome in these cases is shown in Table 9–7, and the time sequence in Table 9–8. In general, the indication for operation has been the finding of severe dysplasia in sequential biopsies, or the presence of severe dysplasia in multiple biopsies obtained on one occasion from various parts of the colon. Under these circumstances, a carcinoma was found in four of seven operation specimens. Operation was delayed if severe dysplasia was an inconstant finding on biopsy, or sometimes if the patient was reluctant to undergo surgical treatment.

Table 9–8 shows that no clear evolution of dysplastic change with time has been discernible in this series. In six patients severe dysplasia was found in the first biopsy, although this was not always a constant finding subsequently. In other patients severe dysplasia was found transiently during follow-up.

Patient C in Table 9–8 is of particular interest because colonoscopic biopsies showed no dysplasia 21 years after the onset of colitis, but when the examination was repeated three years later severe dysplasia was found in four biopsies. Proctocolectomy was undertaken, and there were two ill-defined areas of low polypoid mucosa in the ascending and

TABLE 9-6 Outcome at the End of Follow-up in the 20 Patients in whom One or More Biopsies Showed Moderate Dysplasia

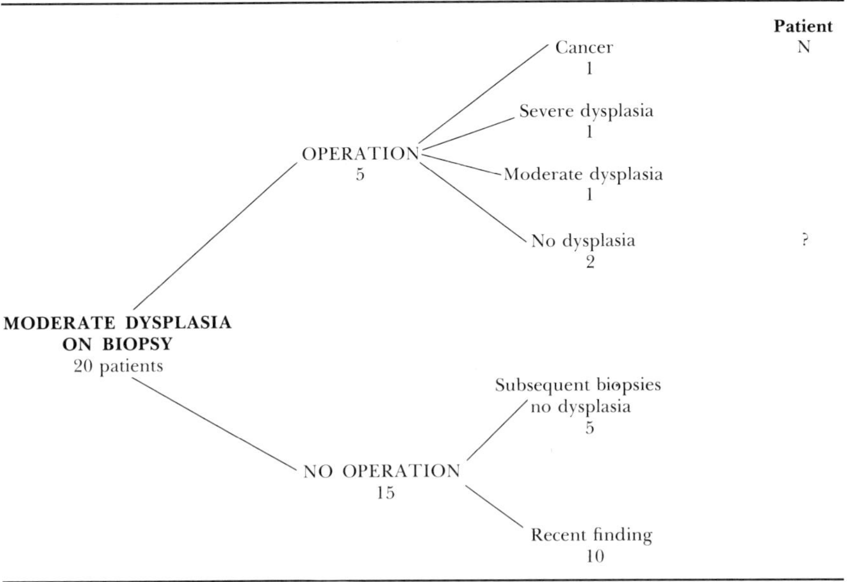

TABLE 9-7 Outcome at the End of Follow-up in the 13 Patients in whom One or More Biopsies Showed Severe Dysplasia

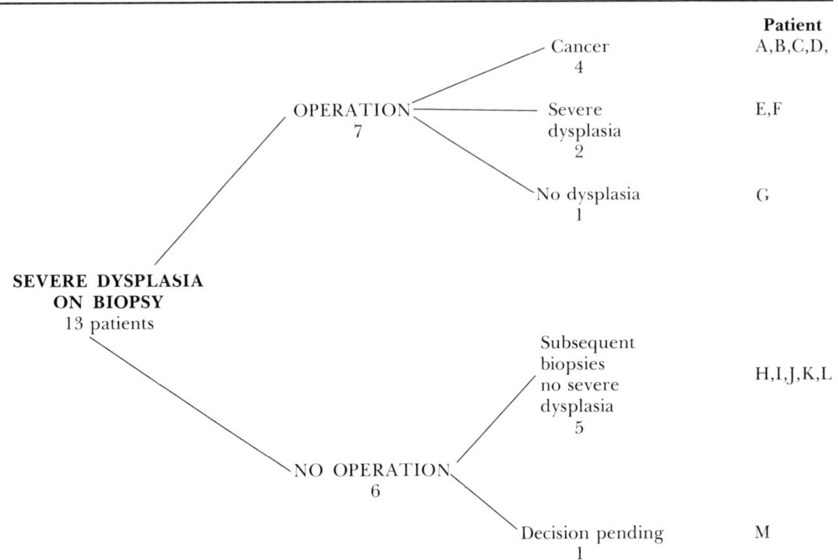

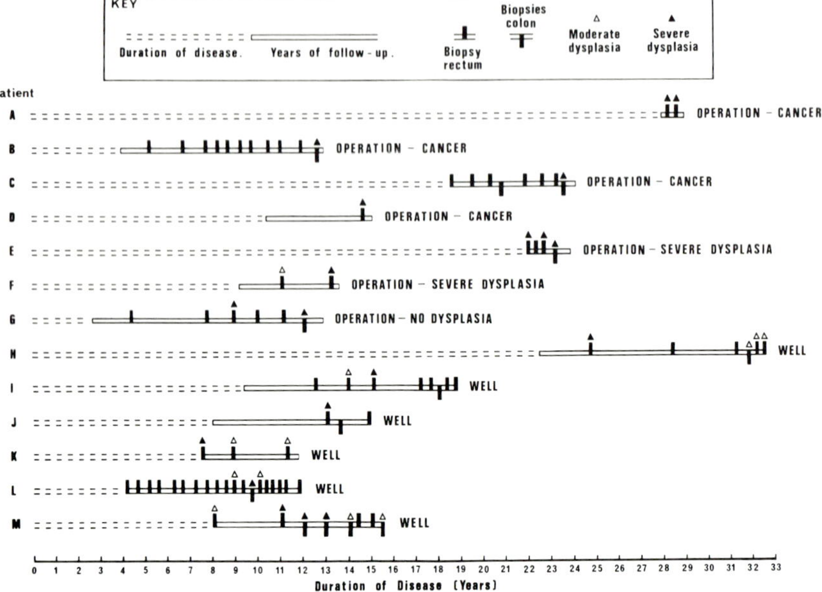

transverse colon. Each of these areas contained a focus of well-differentiated carcinoma with spread limited to the submucosa.

It had been hoped that sequential rectal and colonic biopsies would show that patients passed from a stage of inflammation through a phase of increasing dysplasia before carcinoma developed. In practice it has not been possible to recognize this sequence.

No carcinoma has been detected in which dysplastic changes on biopsy have been absent. It is known that dysplasia can be absent from part or all of the rectum when it is present in the colon (Evans and Pollock, 1972; Myrvold, Kock, and Ahren, 1974; Cook and Goligher, 1975; Riddell, 1976). Our own experience convinces us that multiple biopsies from the colon are necessary to detect dysplasia limited to areas above the reach of the sigmoidoscope. It must also be remembered that carcinoma in colitis has been reported in the absence of significant dysplasia (Evans and Pollock, 1972; Hulten, Kewenter, and Ahren, 1972; Yardley and Keren, 1974; Cook and Goligher, 1975; Riddell, 1976). However, the data do suggest that a patient can be reassured that the short-term risk of carcinoma is very low if severe dysplasia is absent from rectal and colonic biopsies. The finding of moderate dysplasia in a rectal biopsy is an indication for colonoscopy and multiple biopsies, and for increased vigilance in follow-up. If the dysplasia remains mild, or apparently disappears, follow-up should be continued.

Severe dysplasia on biopsy is associated with a high incidence of coincident carcinoma, as has been shown in other studies (Morson and Pang, 1967; Myrvold, Kock, and Ahren, 1974; Yardley and Keren,

1974), but these are early (Dukes A) cancers and the likelihood of cure is high.

The reassurance given by multiple colonic biopsies that show no evidence of dysplasia must necessarily be temporary, but the optimum time interval between examinations has yet to be determined. At present an interval of two years between examinations would appear sufficient, but some authors consider that yearly colonoscopy is advisable (Levin, Riddell, and Kirsner, 1976).

PREVENTION OF CANCER IN COLITIS

Many published studies have shown that the following factors strongly influence the cancer risk in colitis, but none of them is absolute; each increases the probability of developing carcinoma.

(a) *Maximum extent of disease.* The careful study of MacDougall (1964a, b) showed, and other studies have confirmed, that carcinoma generally develops only when colitis has involved most of the large intestine (Edwards and Truelove, 1964; Hinton, 1966; de Dombal et al., 1966), although there are exceptions to this generalization.

(b) *Total length of history.* About 80 per cent of carcinomas in colitis are diagnosed in patients with a total history of ten years or more (Mottet, 1971).

(c) *Age of onset.* There is evidence that colitis beginning in childhood is more likely to be complicated by carcinoma than colitis developing in adult life (Edwards and Truelove, 1964; MacDougall, 1964b; Goldgraber and Kirsner, 1964).

(d) *Epithelial dysplasia.* Several studies of colectomy specimens have shown that severe epithelial dysplasia is usually present at a distance from the tumor when carcinoma complicates colitis, but that the changes are often patchy and can be absent (Morson and Pang, 1967; Evans and Pollock, 1972; Hulten, Kewenter, and Ahren, 1972; Yardley and Keren, 1974; Cook and Goligher, 1975; Riddell, 1976). It is generally agreed that severe dysplasia can be present in the absence of carcinoma.

A program for prevention of cancer in colitis should include the following procedure (Lennard-Jones, Morson, Ritchie, Shove, and Williams, 1977). All patients with extensive colitis, and those in whom the rectum is retained after surgical treatment (Aylett, 1971), need regular follow-up by clinical assessment, sigmoidoscopy, and rectal biopsy. The extent of colitis should be ascertained in all patients by air contrast barium enema. Although colonoscopy with biopsy generally reveals that colitis is more extensive than is shown by radiographs, most published statistics and the data are calculated on the assessment of extent by x-ray examination, and at present this seems the best policy. The radiograph should be repeated if there is clinical suspicion that the area of inflammation has extended.

During the first ten years after onset of colitis, regular sigmoidoscopy and rectal biopsy is preferred to colonoscopy as it is less disturbing for the patient, technically easier, and less expensive. Sigmoidoscopy is likely to detect about 40 per cent of cancers in colitis; dysplasia, when it occurs, involves the rectum in 60 to 80 per cent of cases (Cook and Goligher, 1975; Riddell, 1976). This examination, therefore, appears to be an adequate safeguard at a time when the cancer risk is relatively low.

Once the total length of history exceeds ten years, regular follow-up with sigmoidoscopy should be supplemented by colonoscopy with multiple biopsies every two years, or more frequently if there is a suspicion of dysplasia.

At any stage in follow-up, the finding of possible dysplasia is not an indication for immediate operation. Interpretation can be difficult as the changes of reactive hyperplasia can simulate those of dysplasia (Hulten, Kewenter, and Ahren, 1972; Yardley and Keren, 1974; Riddell, 1976). If, therefore, the biopsy shows evidence of moderate or severe inflammation, it is important to compare the changes in the current biopsy with those of previous and subsequent biopsies. An earlier biopsy showing acute inflammation, but without the suspicious nuclear changes, suggests that these are due to regeneration in the resolving phase of colitis (Morson, 1974). Similarly, a biopsy taken a few weeks later may show that the cytologic abnormalities have disappeared as the colitis becomes inactive (Yardley and Keren, 1974).

Histologic findings should be regarded as an indication for colectomy only if dysplasia is severe, consistent in more than one biopsy obtained at different sites or sequentially or in a single biopsy taken from an endoscopic lesion, and preferably present in the absence of marked inflammation. In a study of 229 patients, only four symptomless patients were advised to undergo colectomy because of the finding of severe dysplasia; three of these were found to have an early carcinoma (Dukes A) (Lennard-Jones, Morson, Ritchie, Shove, and Williams, 1977).

Experience has shown that the follow-up of patients with extensive colitis is demanding in time and resources. Successful follow-up requires a team of workers in different disciplines, all interested in the care of patients with colitis. The clinical staff must establish a relationship of mutual confidence with the patients. The purpose of regular observations (which may be unpleasant and inconvenient) must be explained without causing alarm; analogy with the "cervical smear" is helpful. Clinicians should be aware of the patient's background; for example, a coincidental illness may be a greater risk to life than colitis, and the findings on x-ray examination, endoscopy, and biopsy must be studied. With this knowledge, inconsistencies in the results of investigations may be detected and a balanced decision made about the need for surgical treatment.

Sigmoidoscopy with biopsy is most conveniently performed at each outpatient consultation. Facilities for colonoscopy are also needed. The endoscopist needs to avoid causing the patient discomfort, as repeated examinations are likely, and he should look particularly for any low villous change in the mucosa (although in practice this is difficult to recognize) and biopsy such areas in addition to all parts of the colon.

Since the aim of follow-up is to detect severe dysplasia, or carcinoma at such an early stage that radiologic changes are unlikely, the radiologist's main contributions are to determine the extent of colitis and the configuration of the colon to aid the colonoscopist, and to draw attention to any suspicious areas. The finding of a stricture (Hunt et al., 1975) or large polyp (Teague and Read, 1975) is not diagnostic of carcinoma. Colonoscopy with biopsy or polypectomy is needed to establish the diagnosis.

The pathologist requires experience of the difficulties associated with the recognition of dysplasia in colitis (see Chapter 5). Since severe dysplasia is uncommon, being seen in only 32 of 1,570 biopsies in one series (Lennard-Jones, Morson, Ritchie, Shove, and Williams, 1977), collaboration with other centers in the sharing of material should be encouraged. There is a similar need for conformity in nomenclature, since the same dysplastic biopsy may be called a variety of names, each implying the necessity of colectomy, in different institutions. The importance of close physician-pathologist cooperation cannot be overstressed. The need to interpret a biopsy in the context of earlier and later biopsies has already been emphasized. The continuity of clinical supervision and the collation of data require coordination by a member of staff with responsibility for the administrative aspects of the follow-up.

References

American Cancer Society: Cancer Facts and Figures, 1974.

Aylett, S.: Cancer and ulcerative colitis. Br. Med. J. *2*, 203, 1971.

Cook, M. G., and Goligher, J. C.: Carcinoma and epithelial dysplasia complicating ulcerative colitis. Gastroenterology *68*:1127, 1975.

Crohn, B. B., and Rosenburg, H.: The sigmoidoscopic picture of chronic ulcerative colitis (non-specific). Am. J. Med. Sci. *170*:220, 1925.

Dawson, I. M. P., and Pryse-Davies, J.: The development of carcinoma of the large intestine in ulcerative colitis. Br. J. Surg. *47*:113, 1959.

de Dombal, F. T., Watts, J. M., Watkinson, G., and Goligher, J. C.: Local complications of ulcerative colitis; stricture, pseudopolyposis and carcinoma of colon and rectum. Br. Med. J. *1*:1442, 1966.

Devroede, G. J., Taylor, W. F., Sauer, W. G., Jackman, R. J., and Stickler, G. B.: Cancer risk and life expectancy of children with ulcerative colitis. New Engl. J. Med. *285*:17, 1973.

Dilawari, J. B., Parkinson, C., Riddell, R. H., Loose, H., and Williams, C. B.: Colonoscopy in the investigation of ulcerative colitis. Gut *14*:426, 1973.

Edwards, F. C., and Truelove, S. C.: The course and prognosis of ulcerative colitis: part IV. Gut *5*:15, 1964.

Evans, D. J., and Pollock, D. J.: In-situ and invasive carcinoma of the colon in patients with ulcerative colitis. Gut *13*:566, 1972.

Goldgraber, M. B., and Kirsner, J. B.: Carcinoma of the colon in ulcerative colitis. Cancer *17*:657, 1964.

Goligher, J. C., de Dombal, F. T., Watts, J. McK., Watkinson, G., and Morson, B. C.: Ulcerative Colitis. Balliere, Tindall and Cassell, London, 1968, Chap. 9.

Hinton, J. M.: Risk of malignant change in ulcerative colitis. Gut 7:427, 1966.

Hulten, L., Kewenter, J., and Ahren, C.: Precancer and carcinoma in chronic ulcerative colitis. A histopathological and clinical investigation. Scand. J. Gastroenterol. 7:663, 1972.

Hulten, L., Kewenter, J., and Kock, N. G.: The long-term results of partial resection of the large bowel for intestinal carcinomas complicating ulcerative colitis. Scand. J. Gastroenterol. *6*:601, 1971.

Hunt, R. H., et al.: Colonoscopy in management of colonic strictures. Br. Med. J. *3*:360, 1975.

Lennard-Jones, J. E., et al.: Prospective study of out-patients with extensive colitis. Lancet *1*:1065, 1974.

Lennard-Jones, J. E., Morson, B. C., Ritchie, J. K., Shove, D. C., and Williams, C. B.: Cancer in colitis: assessment of the individual risk by clinical and histological criteria. Gastroenterology, *73*:1280, 1977.

Levin, B., Riddell, R. H., and Kirsner, J. B.: Management of precancerous lesions of the gastrointestinal tract. Clin. Gastroenterol. *5*:827, 1976.

MacDougall, I. P. M.: The cancer risk in ulcerative colitis. Lancet *2*:655, 1964a.

MacDougall, I. P. M.: Clinical identification of those cases of ulcerative colitis most likely to develop cancer of the bowel. Dis. Colon Rectum 7:447, 1964b.

Morson, B. C.: The Technique and Interpretation of Rectal Biopsies in Inflammatory Bowel Disease. *In* Sommers, C. S. (ed.): Pathology Annual. Appleton-Century-Crofts, New York, 1974, pp. 209–230.

Morson, B. C., and Pang, L. S. C.: Rectal biopsy as an aid to cancer control in ulcerative colitis. Gut *8*:423, 1967.

Mottet, N. K.: Histopathologic Spectrum of Regional Enteritis and Ulcerative Colitis. Major Problems in Pathology, Vol. 2. W. B. Saunders Co., Philadelphia, 1971, Chap. 9.

Myrvold, H. E., Kock, N. G., and Ahren, C.: Rectal biopsy and precancer in ulcerative colitis. Gut *15*:301, 1974.

Price, A. B., and Morson, B. C.: Inflammatory bowel disease: the surgical pathology of Crohn's disease and ulcerative colitis. Hum. Pathol. *6*:7, 1975.

Riddell, R. H.: The Precarcinomatous Phase of Ulcerative Colitis. *In* Morson, B. C. (ed.): Topics in Pathology. Springer-Verlag, Berlin, 1976, pp. 179–219.

Rosenqvist, H., Lagercrantz, R., Edling, N., and Ohrling, H.: Ulcerative colitis and carcinoma coli. Lancet *1*:906, 1959.

Svartz, N., and Ernberg, T.: Cancer coli in cases of colitis ulcerosa. Acta Med. Scand. *135*:444, 1949.

Teague, R. H., and Read, A. E.: Polyposis in ulcerative colitis. Gut *16*:792, 1975.

Yardley, J. H., and Keren, D. F.: "Precancer" lesions in ulcerative colitis: a retrospective study of rectal biopsy and colectomy specimens. Cancer *34*:835, 1974.

Yeomans, F. C.: Carcinomatous degeneration of rectal adenoma. J.A.M.A. *89*:852, 1927.

Chapter Ten

The Adenoma-Carcinoma Sequence in the Experimental Animal

J. W. Cole

Much evidence has accumulated, as a result of both basic and clinical research, to suggest that many if not most adenocarcinomas of the colon are the terminal stage in what is frequently referred to as the "polyp-cancer sequence." The evidence, however, remains circumstantial.

Further clarification of this problem is hindered by the fact that in studying any vital process, i.e., a transition from a benign to a malignant state, the methodology available has been inadequate to the task. To date, histopathologists have been limited to describing the appearance of cells and their orientation at a particular point in time, and must make certain assumptions as to changes that may have occurred within a cell or group of cells during the intervals between observations.

Opportunities to study the adenoma-carcinoma sequence in human subjects will continue; however, certain moral and ethical constraints may remain as impediments to this line of investigation.

The recognition that various chemicals [1, 2-dimethylhydrazine (DMH), N-methyl-n′-nitro-N-nitrosoguanidine (MNNG), and 3,2′di-methyl-4-aminobiphenyl (DMABP)] are carcinogenic in laboratory animals, and in some instances nearly colon-specific, has prompted many workers to utilize these experimental models in a study of the adenoma-carcinoma relationship (Walpole et al., 1952; Druckery et al., 1967; Spjut and Noale, 1970; Narisawa et al., 1971).

Thus far the information obtained from these studies is helpful in several respects. Although caution must be exercised in extrapolating the findings to man, the studies have clearly established the fact that both benign adenomas and adenocarcinomas can be induced by a single etiologic agent (Fig. 10–1). A wide variation in morphologic appearance of epithelial tumors is generally found in the same colon, corroborating the view of Morson that villous, adenopapillary, and adenomatous tumors are simply different expressions of the same underlying process (see Chapters 1 and 5).

The experimental observations further suggest that whether an adenocarcinoma develops in the experimental animal or not is, in part, a function of time. Thus, when animals are sacrificed early in the course of administration of the carcinogens, frank cancers are seldom found, but benign adenomas or microscopic foci of abnormal cells can be found on histologic examination. Recent investigations by Felipe (1975) demonstrate the sequential histologic changes in the rat colon that occur following the weekly administration of subcutaneous DMH. In the experimental animals focal hyperplasia of the epithelium could be noted microscopically in the distal colon by the fourth week. "Dysplasia" occurred after a slightly longer period. Carcinoma in situ was not observed until the 15th week, by which time macroscopic lesions were observed. From the 19th week onward, both the size and number of macroscopic lesions increased. Of the 54 macroscopic lesions found between the 19th and 20th weeks, 29 were invasive carcinoma on histologic examination, out of which 79 per cent were located in the distal colon.

Related studies suggest that the chemically induced carcinomas and adenomas in the rat colon are the result of the carcinogenic agent acting on the surface epithelium. The evidence for this derives from the observation that, when a portion of the large bowel was allowed to remain in situ but no longer in contact with the fecal stream, tumors were not observed to occur in the defunctionalized bowel (Navarrete and Spjut, 1967; Cleveland et al., 1967). In other experiments, Narisawa et al. (1971) have reported tumor induction in rats by the intrarectal instillation of carcinogenic agents. Certain carcinogenic compounds, however, may reach the colonic epithelium via the bloodstream.

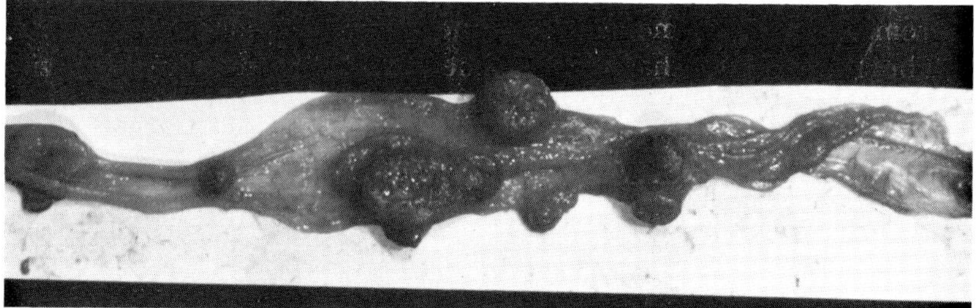

Figure 10–1 Chemically induced (1,2-dimethylhydrazine) (DMH) tumors of the rat colon.

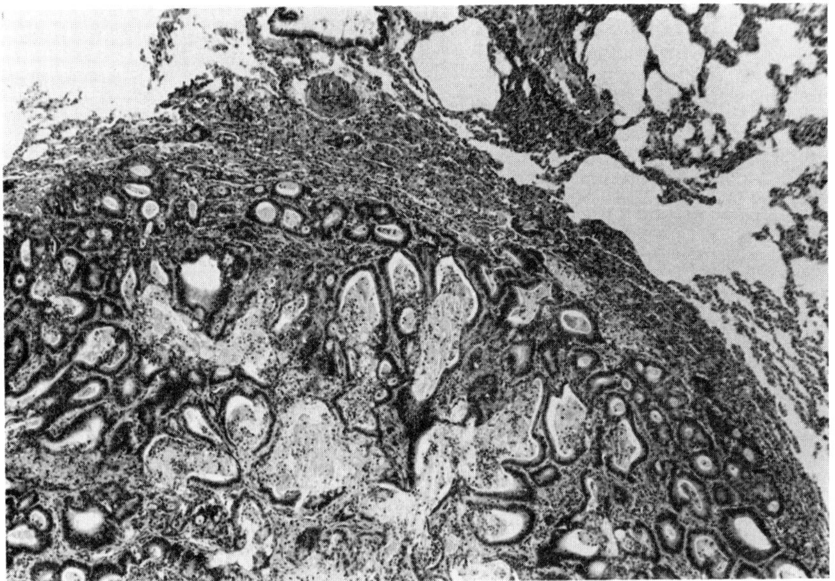

Figure 10–2 Chemically induced (1,2-dimethylhydrazine) (DMH) adenocarcinoma of the colon metastatic to the lung.

Campbell and co-workers (1975), using Sprague-Dawley rats, were able to induce tumors routinely in nonfunctional colon tissue by subcutaneous injection of azoxymethane.

Despite the foregoing observations in experimental animals, the evidence in support of the presumed sequential histologic changes from adenoma to adenocarcinoma remain unclear. However, studies currently in progress will permit direct observation of the tumor by endoscopic or surgical intervention from the time they are first manifest, thus allowing repeated biopsies and histologic evaluation over time. Even with this experimental design, problems in interpretation will remain. The trauma associated with the biopsy procedure itself may alter the tissue in a way that will preclude valid interpretation on subsequent tissue samples of lesions under observation. A further criticism may relate to the possibility, particularly in the larger lesions, that the biopsied specimen may not be representative of the entire lesion. Nonetheless, this approach, now technically feasible, may provide new knowledge about this vexing problem.

Chemically induced tumors in rodents, both benign and malignant, are essentially identical to those found in man, both grossly and microscopically (Spjut and Noale, 1970). In the case of the adenocarcinomas their biologic behavior is comparable. These lesions not only invade adjacent tissue but may metastasize by both lymphatic and hematogenous routes to other organs, i.e., lungs, lymph nodes, and liver (McCall and Cole, 1974). (Figs. 10–2, 10–3, and 10–4).

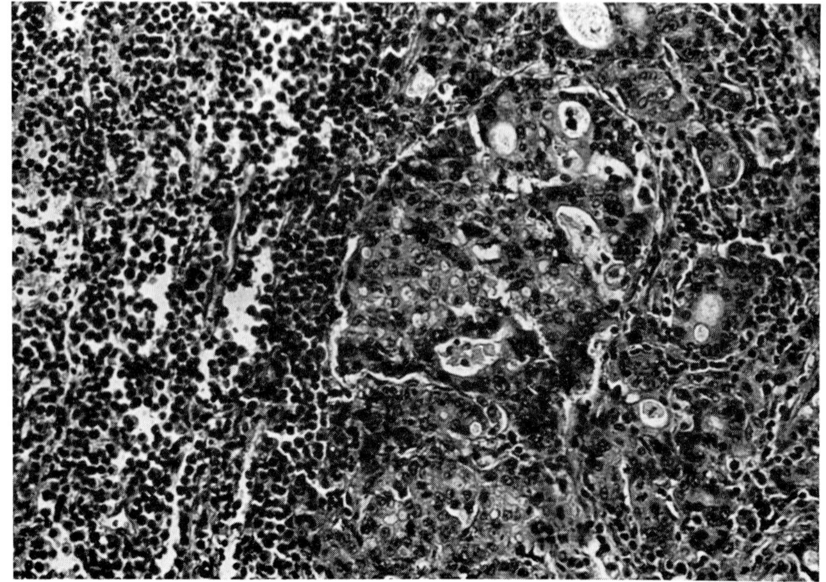

Figure 10–3 Chemically induced (1,2-dimethylhydrazine) (DMH) adenocarcinoma of the colon metastatic to the lymph nodes.

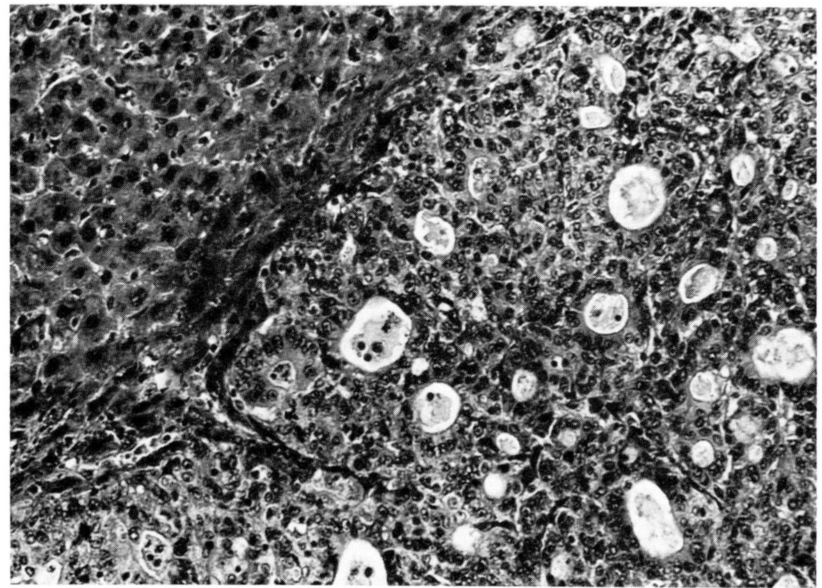

Figure 10–4 Chemically induced (1,2-dimethylhydrazine) (DMH) adenocarcinoma of the colon metastatic to the liver.

Aside from the fact that it has long been established that a variety of chemical compounds can produce colon adenomas and carcinomas in rats, early workers recognized the possible role of bacteria in tumor induction.

Laqueur (1970) showed that a high percentage of rats fed cycasin developed tumors of the large bowel, but when these animals were maintained in a germ-free state, no tumors occurred. It is also of interest to note that cycasin is a naturally occurring carcinogen. More recently several different groups of investigators have pursued this line of investigation, and the results confirm the findings that bacteria are important in tumor induction (Hill et al., 1971).

Reddy and co-workers (1975) found that DMH induced colonic tumors in only 20 per cent of the group of germ-free rats, whereas 93 per cent of the conventional rats developed multiple colonic tumors. In contrast, the number of colon tumors per rat was higher in mono-contaminated and germ-free rats than in the conventional controls following intrarectal administration of azoxymethane. The authors were led to speculate that in the germ-free state absorption of AOM from the gut might be enhanced, resulting in altered metabolism of the compound in the liver with the production of increased levels of co-carcinogens and/or carcinogens reaching the large bowel.

Other factors also appear to be significant in colon carcinogenesis, including bile acids and sterols.

Hill and Aries (1971) studied the fecal composition of four different population groups with regard to steroids and bile pigments. In the English and Scottish group with a high incidence of colon cancer, they found higher concentration of urobilin and acid and neutral steroids, which were more microbially degraded than those in the feces from Ugandans and Indians with a lower incidence of colon cancer.

Additional studies in rats have shown that increasing the bile content of the large bowel by transposition of the bile duct to the midportion of the small intestine enhances the carcinogenic effect of azoxymethane (Chomchai et al., 1974).

Narisawa et al. (1974) have also observed that taurodeoxycholeic acid had a promoting effect on colon carcinogenesis.

Assuming that bile acids and bacteria are contributing factors in colon carcinogenesis, it follows that the composition of ingested foodstuff may also be important since it affects the bacterial flora of the gut as well as the various secretions that are important in the digestive process (Reddy et al., 1974).

The possible relationship between diet and colon carcinogenesis resulted in part from several demographic studies that demonstrated wide variation in the incidence of adenomas and adenocarcinomas of the colon between certain ethnic and racial populations. Examples include the low incidence of colon tumors in black natives of Africa (Bremner and Ackerman, 1970).

It has also been shown that, when populations with a low incidence of colon cancer migrate to countries with a higher incidence and adopt their dietary habits, subsequent generations of offspring manifest the same high incidence of colonic neoplasm as that noted in their adopted country, the most notable example of this being the Japanese. In Japan, the incidence of colon and rectal cancer is quite low. However, the descendants of Japanese immigrants to the United States are known to have colon cancer with a frequency comparable to native-born Americans (Stemmermann, 1970).

Although it is still not clear which of the many foodstuffs included in western-style diets may play a role in this increased incidence, Haenszel and co-workers (1973) have found a close correlation with the ingestion of beef. More refined studies will be required to determine which of the many constituents of beef, if any, to incriminate; however, the fat content is suspect in light of the possible part played by sterols in colon carcinogenesis. For instance, rats maintained on high-fat diets are more susceptible to colon tumor induction by DMH than rats fed a low-fat diet (Reddy et al., 1946).

Other dietary ingredients, however, have been considered during the past several years since Burkitt (1971) first drew attention to the difference in fiber content between the food of African natives with a low incidence of colon cancer and that of whites with a high incidence of colon cancer; the latter group ate highly refined foods that were low in fiber content. He also pointed out how this influenced stool bulk and transit times, which might be important should the carcinogenic agent be exerting its effect by direct contact with a susceptible colonic epithelium.

The complexity of the problem is further appreciated when one considers the wide array of chemical compounds used today in the food processing industry, particularly in the so-called "developed countries" where, in general, the incidence of colon cancer is the highest.

It may be concluded from the foregoing account of the various experimental approaches to the adenoma-carcinoma sequence that the actual "cause" of a neoplastic growth in the colon's epithelium will be multifactorial. Even if future studies make it possible to define more precisely those factors in the environment that conceivably bear on the development of large bowel tumors, we must still understand more fully the difference in individual susceptibility. This must include consideration of possible genetic determinants, immune mechanisms, and the hormonal milieu.

It is clear that our understanding is incomplete of the ultimate alterations that occur within the normal cell to change it from one that has been "programmed" to perform a particular role in support of the body's economy to one that is independent of normal controls and restraints. However, progress is being made, and the experimental evidence continues to suggest that a variety of environmental factors interact to produce neoplastic changes both benign and malignant in the susceptible colonic epithelium.

References

Bremner, C.G., and Ackerman, L.V.: Polyps and carcinoma of the large bowel in South African Bantu. Cancer *26*:991, 1970.

Burkitt, D.P.: Epidemiology of cancer of the colon and rectum. Cancer *28*:3, 1971.

Campbell, R.L., Singh, D.V., and Nigro, N.D.: Importance of the fecal stream on the induction of colon tumors by azoxymethane in rats. Cancer Res. *35*:1369, 1975.

Chomchai, C., Bhadrachari, N., and Nigro, N.D.: The effect of bile on the induction of experimental intestinal tumors in rats. Dis. Colon Rectum *17*:310, 1974.

Cleveland, J.C., Litvak, S.F., and Cole, J.W.: Identification of the route of action of the carcinogen 3,2′-dimethyl-4-aminobiphenyl in the induction of intestinal neoplasia. Cancer Res. *27*:708, 1967.

Druckery, H., Preussmann, R., Matzkies, A., and Ivankovic, S.: Selektive Erzeugung von Darmkrebs bei Ratten durch 1,2-Dimethyl-hydrizin. Naturwissenschaften *54*:285, 1967.

Felipe, M.I.: Mucus secretion in rat colonic mucosa during carcinogenesis induced by dimethylhydrazine. A morphological and histochemical study. Br. J. Cancer *32*:60, 1975.

Haenszel, W., Berg, J., Segi, M., Kurihara, M., and Locke, F.: Large bowel cancer in Hawaiian Japanese. J. Natl. Cancer Inst. *51*:1765, 1973.

Hill, M.J., and Aries, V.C.: Fecal steroid composition and its relationship to cancer of the large bowel. J. Pathol. *104*:129, 1971.

Hill, M.J., Drasar, B.S., Aries, V., Crowther, J.S., Hawsksworth, G., and Williams. R.E.O.: Bacteria and etiology of cancer of the large bowel. Lancet *1*:95, 1971.

Laqueur, G.L.: Contributions of Intestinal Microflora to Carcinogenesis. *In* Burdette, W.J. (ed.): Carcinoma of the Colon and Antecedent Epithelium. Charles C Thomas, Springfield, Ill., 1970, pp. 2051–2313.

McCall, D.C., and Cole, J.W.: Transplantation of chemically induced adenocarcinomas of the colon in an inbred strain of rats. Cancer *33*:1021, 1974.

Narisawa, T., et al.: Promoting effect of bile acids on colon carcinogenesis after intrarectal instillation of N-methyl-N′-nitro-N-nitrosoguanidine in rats. J. Natl. Cancer Inst. *53*:1093, 1974.

Narisawa, I., Sato, T., Hayakawa, M., Sakuma, A., and Nakano, H.: Carcinoma of the colon and rectum of rats by rectal infusion of MNNG. Gann *62*:231, 1971.

Navarrete, A., and Spjut, H.J.: Effect of colostomy on experimentally produced neoplasms of the colon of the rat. Cancer *20*:1466, 1967.

Reddy, B.S., Narisawa, T., Wright, P., Vukersich, D., Weisburger, J.H., and Wynder, E.L.: Colon carcinogenesis with azoxymethane and dimethylhydrazine in germ-free rats. Cancer Res. *35*:387, 1975.

Reddy, B.S., Weisburger, J.H., and Wynder, E.L.: Fecal bacterial β glucoronidase: control by diet. Science *183*:416, 1974.

Reddy, B.S., Weisburger, J.H., and Wynder, E.L.: Effect of dietary fat level and 1,2-dimethylhydrazine on fecal acid and neutral sterol excretion and colon carcinogenesis in rats. J. Natl. Cancer Inst. *52*:507, 1974b.

Spjut, H.J., and Noale, M.W.: Colonic Neoplasms Induced by 3,2′ Dimethyl-4-aminobiphenyl. *In* Burdette, W.J. (ed.): Carcinoma of the Colon and Antecedent Epithelium. Charles C Thomas, Springfield, Ill., 1970, pp. 280–288.

Stemmermann, G.N.: Patterns of disease among Japanese living in Hawaii. Arch. Environ. Health *20*:266, 1970.

Walpole, A.L., Williams, H.C., and Roberts, D.C.: The carcinogenic action of 4-aminobiphenyl and 3,2′ dimethyl-4-aminobyphenyl. Indian Med. Assoc. *9*:255, 1952.

Chapter Eleven

Epidemiology of Polyps and Cancer

Pelayo Correa

In order to examine the polyp-cancer sequence from the epidemiologic point of view, the epidemiology of large bowel cancer will be briefly reviewed and then compared with what we know of the epidemiology of the different types of polyps of the large bowel. The similarities in the epidemiology of both conditions will be used as a basis for drawing inferences as to the polyp-cancer sequence.

REVIEW OF COLORECTAL CANCER EPIDEMIOLOGY

The epidemiology of large bowel cancer has been the subject of several recent reviews (Haenszel and Correa, 1971; Burkitt, 1971; Wynder, 1975). A series of well-established facts have been brought to light, as well as some promising speculations on causal implications which are under current study. The most prominent facts will be mentioned first.

International Variation

There is marked interpopulation variation in the incidence and mortality of large bowel cancer (Haenszel and Correa, 1971). Fig-

Work supported by contract #N01-CP-53521. National Cancer Institute, NIH, USPHS.

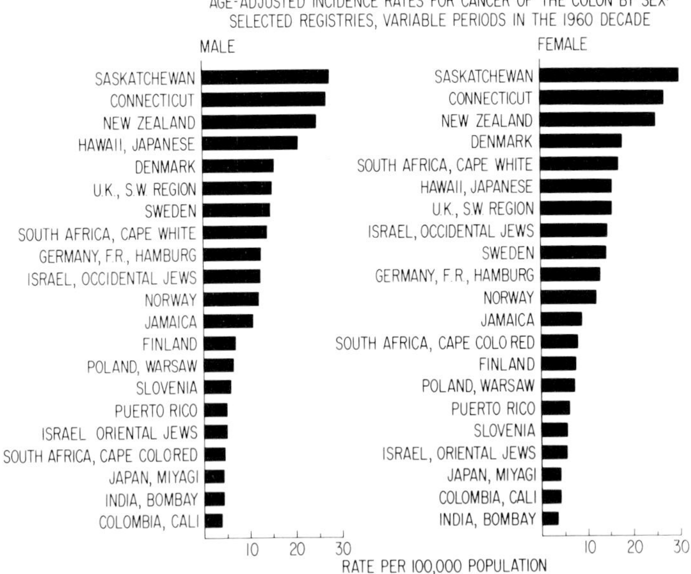

Figure 11–1.

ure 11–1 shows a sevenfold range in age-adjusted incidence rates for colon cancer in selected populations.

Socioeconomic Gradient

With the outstanding exception of Japan, high incidence rates are observed in populations with high socioeconomic standards, whereas low rates are found in populations economically underprivileged.

This socioeconomic gradient is not prominent within populations of high risk (Doll et al., 1970). In populations at low risk, a socioeconomic gradient is detected for cancers arising in the intermediate segments of the colon, but not for those in the cecum or the rectum (Correa, 1975; Haenszel et al., 1975). Table 11–1 shows the stand-

TABLE 11–1 Standardized Incidence Ratio of Large Bowel Cancer by Anatomic Localization and Socioeconomic Class: Cali, Colombia, 1962 to 1971

	Standardized Incidence Ratio Class I + II/III	
Anatomic Localization	*Males*	*Females*
Cecum	0.75	0.94
Ascending through sigmoid	3.92	1.90
Rectum	0.89	1.44

ardized incidence ratios that result from dividing the age-adjusted incidence rates in the upper socioeconomic classes of Cali, Colombia. A different response of the segments of the colon to factors associated with social class is clearly demonstrated in this Table. The incidence of cancer of the intermediate segments of the colon in males is four times greater than the incidence of cancer of the cecum or of the rectum. In females the greater incidence in the intermediate segments of the colon is present but of lesser magnitude.

Human Migration

Migrants from countries where the risk of large bowel cancer is low to countries where such risk is high acquire the high risk of the host country within their lifetime. Figure 11–2 shows that the rates for the first (Issei) and second (Nisei) generation of migrants from Japan to Hawaii are considerably higher than for individuals residing in the country of their birth (Haenszel and Kurihara, 1968). Similar phenomena have been observed in Norwegian migrants to the U.S.A. and Polish migrants to Australia. This increase in incidence seems to take place after the second decade of migration, indicating an incubation period of at least 20 years (Haenszel, 1961; Staszewski and Haenszel, 1965; Haenszel and Kurihara, 1968).

Anatomic Distribution

The excess risk in migrants is first noticed in males, and is concentrated in the sigmoid colon during the initial years of the epidemic (Stemmermann, 1966; Haenszel and Correa, 1971). In populations where a high risk has been documented for several decades, further increases in risk are seen in the more proximal colon segments (transverse, ascending, cecum) (Haenszel and Correa, 1971; Cadey et al., 1974). In such cases, males always show the increased risk earlier and to a greater degree than females. With time, however, rates for females become equal to or higher than those for males.

In low-risk countries, carcinomas of the cecum and ascending colon are more frequent than carcinomas of the left colon. In high-risk countries, on the other hand, sigmoid colon cancers are predominant (Wynder, 1975). Figure 11–3 shows the relative distribution of colon cancer by site in the United States (high-risk) and in Japan (low-risk), demonstrating the relative excess of sigmoid cancer in the U.S. Table 2 illustrates the acceleration of colon cancer in the sigmoid as the total rates for colon cancer increase. In this Table the ratio of cancer of the sigmoid to that of the cecum and ascending colon, and of cancer of the sigmoid to that of the rectum, is shown. The

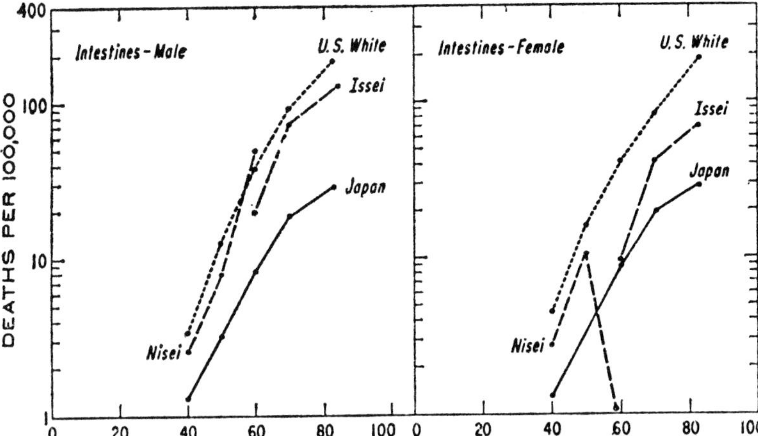

Figure 11–2 Age-specific death rates for intestinal cancers in Japanese-born who migrated to Hawaii (Issei), their Hawaii-born descendants (Nisei), U.S. whites, and Japanese. (*From* Haenszel, W., and Kurihara, M.: J. Natl. Cancer Inst. *40*:43, 1968.)

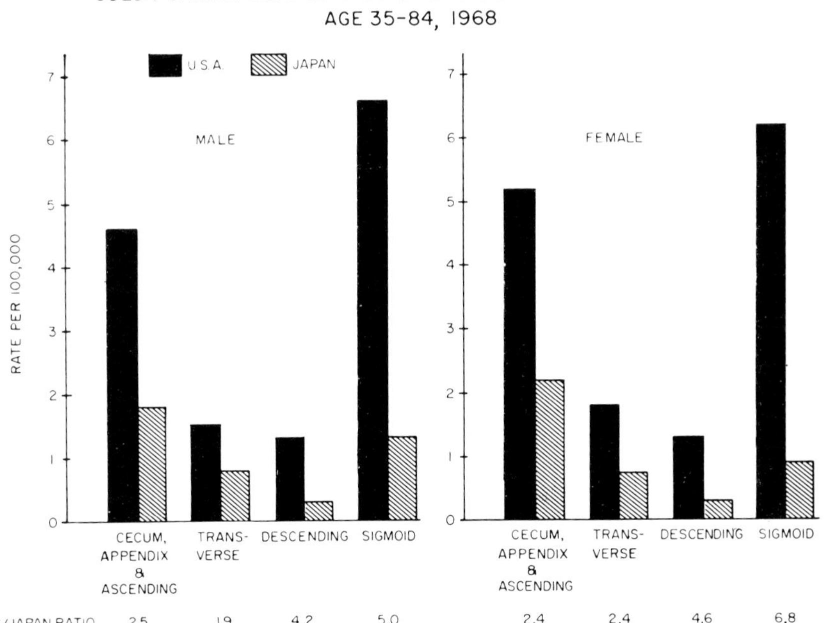

Figure 11–3 (*From* Wynder, E. L.: Cancer Bes. *35*:3388, 1975.)

TABLE 11–2 Cancer Registries Listed in Ascending Order of Total Colon Cancer Incidence

	Colon Cancer Incidence Rate		Males		Females	
	Males	*Females*	*S/C-A*	*S/R*	*S/C-A*	*S/R*
India (Bombay), 1964–1967	4.1	3.4	0.20	0.04	0.33	0.04
Colombia (Cali), 1962–1968	3.6	4.0	0.20	0.10	0.42	0.12
Japan (Miyagi), 1959–61	4.1	4.0	0.41	0.10	0.48	0.14
Puerto Rico, 1950–1968	4.9	6.0	0.71	0.16	0.89	0.28
Finland, 1964–1965	6.8	7.3	0.60	0.16	0.86	0.27
Norway, 1965–1966	12.0	11.6	1.17	0.55	0.92	0.76
Connecticut, 1960–1962	26.7	26.7	1.56	0.68	1.04	0.83

countries are ranked by ascending order of colon cancer risk. It shows the predominance of sigmoid tumors in higher-risk countries.

Colon Rectum Correlation

There is a positive international correlation between incidence rates of cancer of the colon and cancer of the rectum (Haenszel and Correa, 1971). A close scrutiny, however, shows that these two sites differ in other epidemiologic parameters. Figure 11–4 shows that the incidence rates for colon cancer increased in Connecticut from 1940

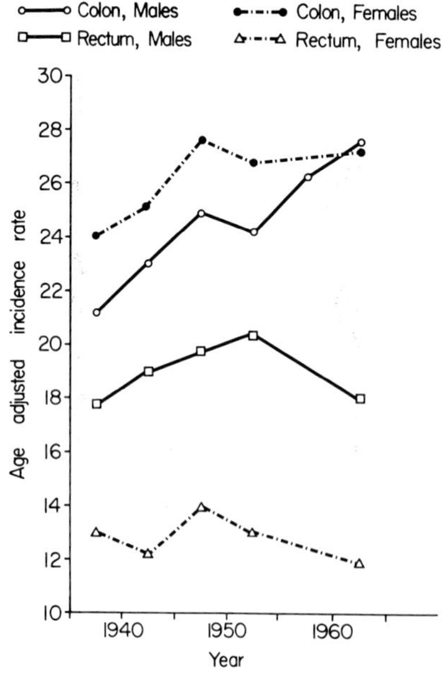

Figure 11–4 Age-adjusted incidence rates for cancer of the colon and rectum by sex, Connecticut, U.S.A. (*From* Axtell, L. M., and Chiazze, L., Jr.: Cancer *19*:750, 1966.)

to 1965, whereas the incidence of rectal cancer remained stable or became slightly lower (Axtell and Chiazze, 1966). The discrepancies between the two observations seem to indicate that rectal cancer comprises two epidemiologic entities at least partially separable by anatomic landmarks (Berg and Haenszel, in preparation). Tumors of the upper rectum have the epidemiologic characteristics of colon cancer, and are excessive in populations where the latter is very frequent. Tumors of the lower rectum do not reflect the fluctuations of colon cancer incidence. Table 11–3 shows an excess of tumors located in the upper rectum in New Orleans (high colon cancer risk) as compared with Cali, Colombia (low colon cancer risk). The New Orleans/Cali ratio is obtained by dividing the proportion of tumors assigned to each anatomic segment in New Orleans by the corresponding proportion in Cali. Tumors of the lower rectum, on the other hand, are excessive in Cali as compared with New Orleans. The positive colon-rectum correlation, therefore, seems to apply to the upper-rectal tumors, whereas lower-rectal tumors probably obey a different set of etiologic factors. The increase in risk of colon cancer observed in some populations of the United States in recent decades has been accompanied by a selective increase in risk of upper-rectal, and a decrease in lower-rectal, cancer. These changes have invalidated the old assertion that most rectal cancer can be found by the examining finger (Berg and Howell, 1974).

Age-Specific Incidence Patterns

Age-specific colon cancer incidence rate curves for males and females cross over some time after the female menopause, and their crossover patterns reflect the level of risk of a community (Haenszel and Correa, 1971). In low-risk countries, represented in Figure 11–5 by Cali, Colombia, female colon cancer rates are higher after menopause. This is the type of curve observed for cancer of the cecum and ascending colon in most countries. In high-risk countries, represented by Connecticut in Figure 11–5, male rates are higher after age 55, a

TABLE 11–3 Relative Distribution of Sigmoid and Rectal Cancer Among Males in New Orleans and in Cali, 1962 to 1972*

Distance from Anus (cm)	Frequency Ratio (New Orleans/Cali)
16+	1.7
6–15	1.2
2–5	0.5
0–1	0.3

**From* Correa, P.: Cancer Res. *35*:3395, 1975.

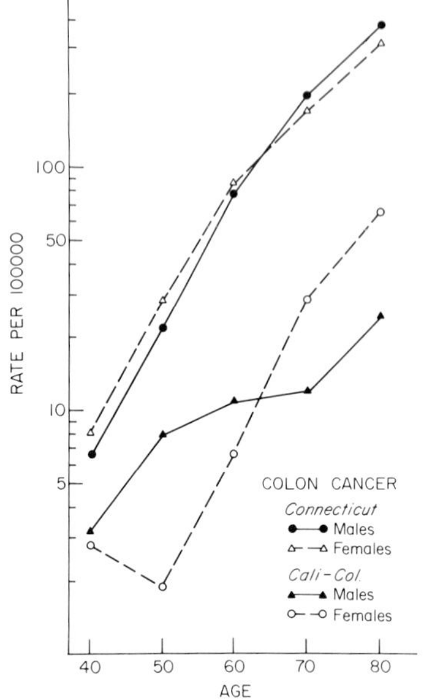

Figure 11-5 Age-specific incidence rates for colon and rectum cancer in Connecticut, U.S.A. (1963–65) and Cali, Colombia (1962–66). (*From* Haenszel, W., and Correa, P.: Dis. Colon Rectum *16*:371, 1973.)

pattern observed in most countries for sigmoid cancer. It seems, therefore, that the age-specific incidence pattern of colon cancer is dominated by the cecum in low-risk countries and by the sigmoid in high-risk countries.

Epidemiologic Model

The above observations have led to the proposal of the following model of colon cancer epidemiology (Haenszel and Correa, 1971):

1. In low-risk populations where the disease is "endemic," colon cancers are concentrated in the cecum and ascending colon. Colon cancer is preponderant in females, and most of the rise to the maximum incidence level has occurred by age 50 to 55.

2. When a new etiologic factor is introduced into such a population, the transition from an "endemic" to an "epidemic" phase is first expressed as a rise in sigmoid cancers among men over 55 years.

3. A rise in female sigmoid cancer occurs later, and the time lag is reinforced by a tendency for these cancers to appear at somewhat older ages than in males.

4. As exposures to the etiologic factor become more intense and prolonged, a later phase is characterized by a rise in cecum and ascending colon cancer. This rise is more marked for males than females, and tends to diminish or obliterate the female excess in cecum cancers prevailing under "endemic" conditions. The changes

for cecum and ascending colon cancer are accompanied by similar transitions in the transverse and descending colon, so that the upward displacement in cases of colon cancer in males may appear sequentially in time as involving successive segments of the colon moving from the rectosigmoid junction to the cecum.

The dynamics of the epidemic type of colon cancer can be explained by the action of an environmental carcinogen in the intestinal content that becomes more concentrated, more potent, or more effective as it travels from the cecum to the rectosigmoid area. Since the epidemic type of colon cancer is correlated with changes in the diet (Haenszel and Berg, 1973) it seems logical to infer that such carcinogen is related to the diet of "western" populations with high socioeconomic standards. However, no carcinogen has been convincingly demonstrated in such diets. The distal position of the colonic mucosa in the gastrointestinal tract makes it likely that an ingested carcinogen would either produce its effects in upper portions of the tract, or be substantially modified before it reaches the colonic mucosa.

Diets of populations at very different colon cancer risk contrast mainly in the following items.

BULK

High-residue diets generally prevail in countries where colon cancer is not frequent. It has been speculated that the faster transit time associated with such diets prevents the action of a carcinogen present in the lumen (Burkitt, 1971). Other studies have failed to corroborate an association between transit time, amount of undigestible fiber in the diet, and colon cancer risk. Colon cancer risk is elevated when ingestion of legumes, with high fiber content, is high (Burkitt, 1971). Experimental studies have failed to detect a strong effect of dietary bulk on colon cancer incidence (Ward et al., 1973). Although the effect of undigestible fibers on colon cancer frequency is not settled, the observations in human populations remain valid; however, the effect is not large enough to explain by itself the present epidemic of the wealthy western countries. With or without the absorbent effects of undigestible fibers, the consensus is that a carcinogen is present in the intestinal content, and efforts to find it will undoubtedly continue.

FAT

There is a good correlation between the amount of fat in the diet and the risk of colon cancer (Wynder, 1975). It has been proposed that high fat intake leads to greater production of cholesterol and cholesterol metabolites that may be carcinogenic (Wynder, 1975). Blood cholesterol levels in colon cancer patients, however, tend to be lower instead of higher (Rose et al., 1974). Correlations with such cholesterol-linked disease as myocardial infarction are positive (Haenszel et al., 1975) but this is to be expected since both diseases are positively correlated with higher socioeconomic standards. More work is needed before deciding whether the association with fat intake is causal.

MEAT

Meat is the dietary item showing the best correlation with colon cancer risk. This has been observed in different populations on the basis of food consumption and mortality rates. In Argentina, with a very high meat consumption, colon cancer rates are as high as those of the United States (Puffer and Griffith, 1967). The positive correlation with meat has also been found in case-control studies (Haenszel and Berg, 1973) and in social class correlations (Correa, 1975).

Bacterial Flora

The above diet peculiarities most probably account for the great interpopulation differences that have been found in the composition of the bacterial flora. Feces from people in Britain and the United States have higher counts of bacteroides and lower counts of enterococci and other anaerobic bacteria than feces from people of Uganda, South India, or Japan, where colon cancer is of low frequency (Hill et al., 1971). Some species of clostridia have been reported to be of excessive frequency in patients with colon cancer (Hill et al., 1971; Hill, 1974), but this finding has not been confirmed in subsequent studies (Finegold et al., 1975; Moore and Holdeman, 1975).

The role of bacteria in colon carcinogenesis is thought to be related to the effect on the degradation products of certain chemical compounds found in the intestinal content. Such a mechanism would fit very well the epidemiologic model, since it would result in cumulatively greater amounts of carcinogen being delivered to the intestinal content from cecum to rectosigmoid. This assumption has found abundant experimental support in the studies of carcinogenic effects of cycasin. This compound, not carcinogenic in itself, is metabolized to methylazoximethanol (MAM) by the intestinal flora. Colon cancer is induced in experimental animals by feeding cycasin, but its occurrence is prevented when the action of the intestinal flora is suppressed by use of germ-free animals or surgical bypass of the fecal stream (Cole, 1969; Laqueur, 1970; Gennaro et al., 1973). In humans, the prime suspects for precarcinogenic substrates are the steroids. Their concentration in the intestinal content is greatly influenced by the ingestion of fat. Feces of people from western countries have a greater concentration of steroids than those of African or Oriental countries (Hill et al., 1971).

In the former countries the steroids are more degraded, raising the possibility that some metabolic products have a carcinogenic effect. Acid steroid (from bile secretions) and neutral steroids (diet-dependent) may be modified by intestinal bacteria; this possibility is under study at the present time, but no definite proof of this etiologic hypothesis is still available. Of interest is the preliminary report by Bone et al. (1975), which shows that patients with familial polyposis do not transform their fecal cholesterol to its metabolites coprostanol and coprostanone, in spite of the presence of bacteria with that capability in their intestinal content. If confirmed, these findings introduce the possibility of explaining colon cancer on the basis of the inability of bacteria to degrade neutral steroids. This inability could be brought about by the absence of such bacteria in the intestinal lumen, or by the inhibition of their degrading function by chemical substances or by other bacteria. The work of Wilkins failed to confirm the presumptive role of neutral steroid degradation in polyp-bearing patients. In short, current thinking of colon cancer epidemiology is concentrating on in situ bacterial synthesis of carcinogens influenced by diet-determined alteration in the microenvironment of the colon.

THE EPIDEMIOLOGY OF POLYPS

We will deal in this section with the descriptive epidemiology of juvenile, hyperplastic, and adenomatous polyps. In the latter category are included adenomatous polyps with villous changes ("tubulovillous adenomas"). Pure villous adenomas are not reviewed because of the scarcity of epidemiologic data available. Our emphasis is on environmental epidemiology, and no attempt is made to review such genetically determined entities as familial polyposis. Gardner's syndrome, or Peutz-Jeghers syndrome.

Juvenile Polyps

Most of the claims of a malignant potential for juvenile polyps date back to the time when their distinction from adenomatous polyps, familial polyposis, villous adenoma, and Peutz-Jeghers polyps was not well-documented. The prevalence of juvenile polyps is summarized in Table 11–4, which shows data for three different series, two from autopsies and one from surgical pathology material. These polyps are rare during the first year of life; their prevalence is highest from 1 to 7 years of age and drops sharply after adolescence, being infrequent in adults. They are more frequent in boys than in girls,

TABLE 11-4 Distribution of Juvenile Polyps by Age and Sex

Autopsies – Colombia*				Autopsies – U.S.A.†				Surgical Pathology AFIP – USA‡	
Age	*Number of Specimens*		*Prevalence Rate*	*Age*	*Number of Specimens*		*Prevalence Rate*	*Age*	*Number of Cases*
0–14	Males	208	6.3	0–1	Males	161	0	0–1	1
	Females	170	2.9		Females	123	0	1–4	58
								5–9	39
15–44	Males	348	3.5	1–10	Males	56	5.3	10–14	1
	Females	209	3.4		Females	29	0	15–19	17
								20–24	19
45–64	Males	279	1.4	11–20	Males	49	0	25–29	8
	Females	95	1.0		Females	31	6.4	30–35	8
								35+	7
65+	Males	126	0.8					Total boys 0–10 years	62
	Females	59	0						
								Total girls 0–10 years	37
								Total males 11+ years	55
								Total females 11+ years	4

*From Correa, P., et al.: Int. J. Cancer *9*:86, 1972.
†*From* Helwig, E. B.: Am. J. Dis. Child *72*:289, 1946.
‡*From* Roth, S. I., and Helwig, E. B.: Cancer *16*:468, 1963.

and more often single than multiple. Since most of these polyps are not resected, their low-prevalence rate in adults indicates that they are self-amputated or regress spontaneously, well-known events in this condition (Andren and Frieberg, 1956; Roth and Helwig, 1963). Their over-all prevalence (both sexes combined) seems to vary from around 1 per cent in autopsy series from the United States (Helwig, 1946) to around 5 per cent in Colombia (Correa et al., 1972). Although there are not many autopsy series to compare, the above data indicate that the prevalence is higher where colon cancer is less frequent. Reports of surgical series indicate an excess of polyps (70 per cent) located in the rectum. Autopsy series show that they are rather evenly distributed in all the large bowel segments, with some concentration in the rectum (Correa et al., 1972). Table 11–5 compares the findings of a surgical pathology series in the United States (Roth and Helwig, 1963) with an autopsy series in Colombia (Correa et al., 1972) and points out the difference in the location already mentioned for both kinds of series.

From the scarce epidemiologic data available it is still possible to infer that these lesions are mediated by noncongenital environmental factors, operating selectively or exclusively during childhood, which are apparently not related to the causation of large bowel cancer.

Hyperplastic Polyps

Most investigators of the role of hyperplastic polyps have concluded, mainly on morphologic grounds, that they are not precancerous (Morson, 1962; Lane et al., 1971). Some studies, mainly on the basis of interpopulation comparisons of frequency and anatomic distribution, have raised the question that hyperplastic polyps may play a role in large bowel carcinogenesis (Stemmermann and Yatani, 1973).

TABLE 11–5 Location of Juvenile Polyps

	AFIP* Surgical Pathology %	Cali† Autopsies %
Cecum	0.6	9.3
Ascending	1.2	14.8
Transverse	3.6	20.4
Descending	2.4	9.3
Sigmoid	11.0	18.5
Rectum	72.0	27.8
Unspecified	7.8	–
Number of polyps	166	54

*From Roth, S. I., and Helwig, E. B.: Cancer *16*:468, 1963.
†From Correa, P., et al.: Int. J. Cancer *9*:86, 1972.

Detailed autopsy studies have recently become available which allow us to examine this question within an epidemiologic context. Following previously published methodology (Correa et al., 1972), large bowel specimens from a number of countries were examined with the aid of an illuminated magnifying lens, and all mucosal elevations examined microscopically. The investigators participating in these studies have all used the same gross technique, and follow the same histologic criteria for classification of polyps. Table 11–6 summarizes the results of these studies. The populations have been ranked with respect to colorectal cancer frequency, based on the following information. Incidence rates of colon cancer are known for some of them (Doll et al, 1970). Hawaiian-Japanese incidence rates per 100,000 population are 20.7 for males and 15.3 for females. The equivalent rates for Cali, Colombia are 3.6 for males and 4.0 for females; for the population of Miyagi, Japan they are 4.1 for males and 4.0 for females. A four- to fivefold difference in incidence between these groups is clearly established. Recent incidence data are not directly available for New Orleans, but it has been reported that the risk for southern U.S. cities has increased in recent decades (Cutler and Young, 1975). These rates are still lower than those of northern cities but are now approaching the national average. Data for Akita prefecture in Japan are higher than those of Miyagi, and represent the highest rate for Japan (Sato et al., 1976). However, they are regarded as intermediate for the purpose of this publication. The same applies to the rates in São Paulo, following the findings of the inter-American investigation of mortality (Puffer and Griffith, 1967). Low mortality rates have been documented for Costa Rica (Moya de Madrigal, 1974). The Table shows that the population with the highest colorectal cancer frequencies, namely Hawaiian-Japanese, also displays the highest prevalence of hyperplastic polyps, whereas populations of low colorectal cancer risk such as Japan and Costa Rica have very low polyp prevalence rates.

The correlation between the two conditions, however, has many inconsistencies. There is a three- to fourfold difference in prevalence of hyperplastic polyps between Hawaii and New Orleans males, but the cancer incidence rates are only slightly higher (around 1.3 times) in Hawaii than in southern U.S. cities (Doll et al, 1970; Cutler and Young, 1975). The difference in colorectal cancer mortality between Akita and Miyagi prefectures is not reflected in different rates of hyperplastic polyps. The prevalence of hyperplastic polyps, but not the cancer incidence, differs between Japan and Colombia. The data from Table 11–6, therefore, cannot be taken as supporting strongly a premalignant role for hyperplastic polyps. The wide range of intercountry variation in polyp prevalence, and the differences between migrants and nonmigrant Japanese, implicate environmental factors in the causation of hyperplastic polyps. Such factors seem to be

TABLE 11–6 Prevalence of Hyperplastic Polyps

Population	Colon Cancer Frequency	No. of Specimens, Age 20–39	No. of Specimens, Age 40–59	No. of Specimens, Age 60+	Prevalence Rate (%), Age 20–39	Prevalence Rate (%), Age 40–59	Prevalence Rate (%), Age 60+
Males							
Hawaiian-Japanese	Very High	2	26	95	50	69	84
New Orleans White	High	18	67	45	11	19	13
New Orleans Black	High	21	65	132	10	18	14
Brazil (São Paulo)	Intermediate	97	100	100	14	26	40
Japan (Akita)	Intermediate	24	52	93	0	2	2
Japan (Miyagi)	Low	127	184	185	1	2	2
Costa Rica (San Jose)	Low	42	105	176	0	7	7
Colombia (Cali)	Low	241	258	198	6	14	11
Females							
Hawaiian-Japanese	Very High	1	7	68	0	57	73
New Orleans White	High	0	20	23	–	25	30
New Orleans Black	High	18	59	101	6	7	9
Brazil (São Paulo)	Intermediate	100	100	100	12	23	31
Japan (Akita)	Intermediate	8	40	62	0	2	8
Japan (Miyagi)	Low	78	116	127	0	0	3
Costa Rica (San Jose)	Low	42	89	138	5	1	9
Colombia (Cali)	Low	142	96	79	2	9	16

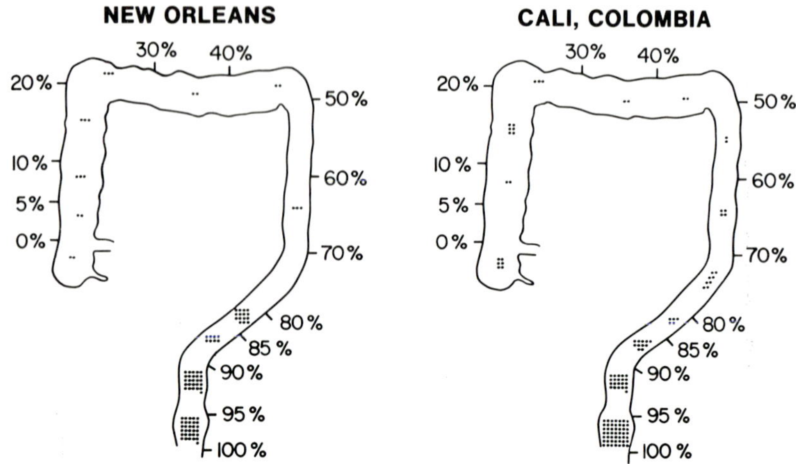

Figure 11–6 Diagrammatic representation of the distribution of hyperplastic polyps in males of New Orleans, U.S.A. (whites and blacks) and Cali, Colombia.

independent from those associated with colorectal cancer. Factors leading to hyperplastic polyps and factors leading to cancer seem to coincide in some populations but not in others.

The anatomic localization of hyperplastic polyps is characterized by its concentration in the rectum and lower sigmoid, with predilection for the lower rectum. Figure 11–6 is a diagrammatic representation of the localization of hyperplastic polyps in New Orleans, where colorectal cancer is very frequent, and in Cali, Colombia, where such tumors are infrequent. In spite of marked differences in colorectal cancer frequency, the difference in prevalence of hyperplastic polyps in the two populations is small (Table 11–6) and the localization shows the same pattern. The same concentration in the more distal segments of the intestine has been found in all the reported series known to the author (Arthur, 1968; Stemmermann and Yatani, 1973; Sato et al., 1976; Marigo; Restrepo; Segura). This anatomic distribution is not congruent with the distribution of the epidemic type of colon cancer, which shows a predominance of the intermediate segments of the colon (Haenszel and Correa, 1971). Such polyp distribution would be more congruent with lower-rectal cancer. Unfortunately, not much is known about the epidemiology of lower-rectal cancer to enable us to draw any firm conclusions concerning its relationship with hyperplastic polyps. Cancer of the rectum in Japan is predominantly localized in the lower segment (Berg and Howell, 1974). The low frequency of hyperplastic polyps in Japan, therefore, argues against a premalignant role for hyperplastic polyps. Lower-rectal cancer is relatively more frequent in Cali than in New Orleans (Correa, 1975), whereas hyperplastic polyps are slightly more prevalent in New Orleans. Thus, the epidemiologic data available at the present time fail to support a premalignant role for hyperplastic polyps.

Adenomatous Polyps

The morphology of the polyp-cancer sequence of adenomatous polyps can be adequately studied in surgical material, but the epidemiology of such sequence is better studied on the basis of the prevalence of both conditions, which cannot be adequately judged from patients in whom polyps are found by the endoscopists or the surgeon. Such patients with adenomatous polyps and/or colon cancer represent index cases and do not give an idea of the size of the population from which they are drawn. The prevalence is given by the number of patients bearing the lesion divided by the population "at risk." Since it is practically impossible to determine the exact frequency of polyps in a living population, we must resort to a study of the autopsy "population" to determine the prevalence of polyps. This allows us to investigate the polyp-cancer sequence following classical epidemiologic steps, which in our case would direct us to seek answers to the following questions:

1. Is there a statistical association between adenomatous polyps and cancer of the large bowel?
2. Is this association consistent with respect to time, geography, and anatomic and demographic variables?
3. Is this association strong?
4. Is this association biologically sound? Are there other nonepidemiologic scientific facts to support the association?
5. Is the association directly causal (one following the other) or indirectly causal (both being effects of a third cause)?

STATISTICAL ASSOCIATION: GEOGRAPHY

The answer to the first question is given by Table 11–7, utilizing data from the same sources as Table 11–6, which gives a reasonable assurance of comparability. The number of specimens examined for each sex and age-group is given in Table 11–6. Table 11–7 shows a good correlation between colon cancer risk and the prevalence of adenomatous polyps in the populations under study, indicating that both lesions are statistically associated. The Hawaiian-Japanese display the highest rates for both lesions, followed by the New Orleans populations. All four populations with low cancer risk also have low polyp prevalence. Akita and São Paulo populations have intermediate rates of both conditions. This association allows geographic groupings

TABLE 11-7 Prevalence of Adenomatous Polyps

Population	Colon Cancer Frequency	Prevalence Rate (%) Age 20–39	40–59	60+
Males				
Hawaiian-Japanese	Very High	50	69	64
New Orleans White	High	0	39	47
New Orleans Black	High	19	26	52
Brazil (São-Paulo)	Intermediate	5	14	30
Japan (Akita)	Intermediate	21	31	46
Japan (Miyagi)	Low	1	9	23
Costa Rica (San Jose)	Low	0	6	13
Colombia (Cali)	Low	2	7	18
Females				
Hawaiian-Japanese	Very High	0	71	58
New Orleans White	High	0	10	35
New Orleans Black	High	0	27	41
Brazil (São-Paulo)	Intermediate	8	14	23
Japan (Akita)	Intermediate	0	8	37
Japan (Miyagi)	Low	4	9	17
Costa Rica (San Jose)	Low	2	4	9
Colombia (Cali)	Low	2	10	15

that are consistent with what we know of colon cancer epidemiology, namely, high risk in the wealthy "western" societies and low risk in Japan and Latin America. The prevalence rate of adenomatous polyps is very similar for males and females within each population, as is the case for colon cancer. The slightly higher polyp prevalence rates observed for males in some populations such as New Orleans are consistent with earlier increases in male rates observed in the initial periods of a colon cancer epidemic (Haenszel and Correa, 1971).

Race

Racial origin by itself does not seem to be an overriding determinant of colon cancer. The Japanese have low rates in their home country and acquire very high rates after migration to Hawaii or California. African blacks have very low incidence (Burkitt, 1971), whereas American blacks have very high incidence rates at the present time (Cutler and Young, 1975). The same type of observations have been made with respect to adenomatous polyps, of which none were found in a series of 14,000 autopsies of South African Bantu reported by Bremner and Ackerman (1970). Williams and co-workers (1975) found only one adenomatous polyp in 40 intestinal polyps surgically removed in Ibadan, Nigeria, compared with 65 adenomatous polyps in 83 polyps surgically removed from blacks living in

Washington, D.C., U.S.A. Blacks living in New Orleans show a prevalence rate for adenomatous polyps which is slightly higher than the rates observed in whites of the same city (Table 11–7).

TIME TRENDS

Time trends are better known for colon cancer than they are for polyps. As shown in Figure 11–3, an increase in cancer incidence has been documented in the United States since 1940 (Axtell and Chlazze, 1966). A series of independent autopsy studies have been made in the United States since 1946, when the prevalence of "adenomas" was reported by Helwig (1947). Although there are differences in methodology between the studies reported in Table 11–8, a general comparison of prevalence in the 40s, 60s, and 70s is possible (Blatt, 1961; Arminski and McLean, 1964; Stemmermann and Yatani, 1973). The Table shows a steady increase in the prevalence of polyps in different locations in the U.S. with time. The rates for New Orleans in the 70s are in the same range as those found in the 60s in the northern cities. This correlates with a somewhat higher incidence rate in the north than in the south reported by the 1969–1971 National Cancer Survey (Cutler and Young, 1975); for instance, that study showed a rate of 35.5 for Pittsburgh, Pennsylvania and 21.2 for Birmingham, Alabama. The data, therefore, showed that the time trends are similar for colon cancer and for adenomatous polyps.

The time trends in the frequency of colon cancer and adenomatous polyps in American blacks have shown even more dramatic changes than those observed in whites. There are no data available for a "perfect" comparison of rates in two different time periods, but some approximation to the real picture is possible with the available data shown in Table 11–9. The incidence rates for colon cancer in blacks in the United States has doubled between the last two National Cancer Surveys, during which time the rates for whites have increased by approximately 15 per cent (Cutler and Devesa, 1973). The increase in prevalence of polyps (St. Louis-New Orleans) during the last 30 years has been sixfold in blacks, and has doubled in whites. The differences are of such magnitude that the observed greater frequency in blacks is very likely significant.

SOCIOECONOMIC GRADIENT

The frequencies of adenomatous polyps and colon cancer tend to run parallel with respect to socioeconomic class. Table 11–10 shows a socioeconomic gradient of similar magnitude for both adenomatous polyps and cancer of the colon in patients of different socioeconomic classes.

TABLE 11–8 Prevalence of Adenomatous Polyps in the United States

Author	*City*	*Year*	Males *20–39*	Males *40–59*	Males *60+*	Females *20–39*	Females *40–59*	Females *60+*
Helwig*	St. Louis, Mo.***	1947	6	14	24	3	11	18
Blatt**	New Rochelle, N.Y.	1961	0	38	51	0	22	42
Arminski	Detroit, Michigan	1964	27	21	43	16	28	36
Correa	New Orleans, La.***	1975	0	39	47	0	10	35
Stemmermann	Honolulu, Hawaii	1972	50	69	64	6	71	58

*Age-groups 21–40; 41–60; 61+.
**Age-groups 30–39; 40–59; 60+.
***Whites only.

TABLE 11–9 Relative Changes in Cancer Incidence* and Polyp Prevalence in the United States

	Percentage Change		
	Cancer Incidence		*Polyp Prevalence*
	1937–1947	*1947–1969*	*1947–1975*
White males	+17	+27	+125
White females	+16	−1	+175
Black males	+5	+90	+566
Black females	+37	+129	+633

**From* Cutler, S. J., and Devesa, S. S.: IARC Scientific Publication, No. 7, Lyon, 1973.

ANATOMIC LOCALIZATION

The anatomic localization of polyps in the colon is shown in Figure 11–7, which presents diagrammatically the distribution of adenomatous polyps in whites and blacks living in New Orleans. The more marked concentration of polyps in the intermediate segments of the colon (ascending to sigmoid) is similar to the distribution of the epidemic type of colon cancer. The distribution is similar to that found in Cali, Colombia (Correa et al., 1972), except that a somewhat greater concentration of polyps is found in the upper rectum and sigmoid colon in patients of both sexes and both races in New Orleans. In the latter city, 17.5 per cent of large bowel adenomatous polyps (80/464) were located between 10 and 22 cm from the anorectal junction. The corresponding figure for Cali is 10 per cent (17/168). This greater concentration of adenomatous polyps in the sigmoid area is very similar to the greater frequency of cancer in the sigmoid area in patients in New Orleans as compared with those in Cali (Table 11–3).

Interpopulation comparisons of the segmental localization of polyps are difficult because the distribution of polyps is age-dependent. Blatt (1961) found that, in patients between 50 and 60 years of age, the sigmoid is the most prevalent site, whereas from 60 to 80 years the ascending colon is the most prevalent site. This indicates a certain degree of variability in the concentration of polyps in the

TABLE 11–10 Social Class Gradient for Cancer and Adenomatous Polyps of the Large Bowel Cali, Colombia, 1962–1971

Socioeconomic Class	Cancer SIR*	Polyp Prevalence (%)
I + II (high)	145	19.8
III	92	13.1
IV (low)	29	4.4

*SIR = Standardized Incidence Ratio. (*From* Haenszel W., et al.: J. Natl. Cancer Inst., *54*:1031, 1975.)

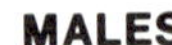

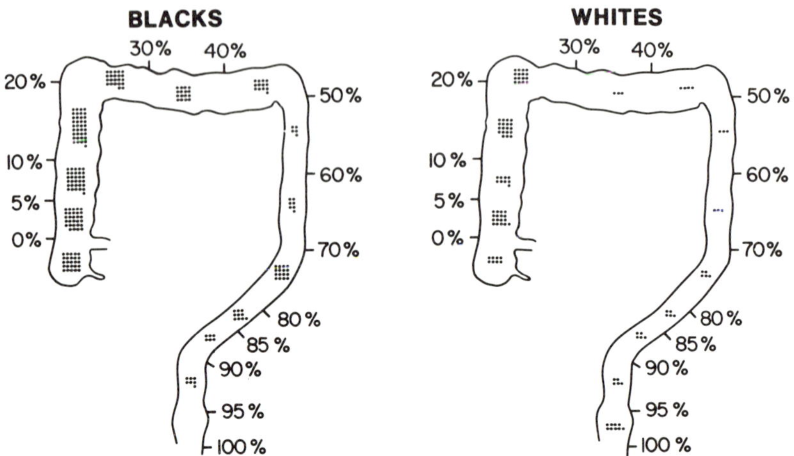

Figure 11-7 Diagrammatic representation of the distribution of adenomatous polyps in white and black males of New Orleans, U.S.A.

different groups in a population, thus making international comparisons difficult without age-matched populations.

If polyp-producing dietary factors are introduced in a community, the duration and intensity of the exposure will vary with the age of each individual (cohort effect). An autopsy sample including persons of different ages represents a cross-section of the population that may not show the cohort effects of such environmental factors.

STRENGTH OF THE ASSOCIATION

The strength of the association is usually evaluated by searching for the equivalent of a dose response, in the sense that an increase in the "dose" (greater amount, greater size, greater number) results in an increase of the effect (more pronounced, more frequent). We should determine, therefore, whether or not an increase in the size or the number of polyps in polyp-bearers correlates with an increased risk of cancer. Table 11-11 gives information on the size of polyps in

TABLE 11-11 Average Size (mm) of Adenomatous Polyps by Age and Location

	Age			
	15-44	*45-54*	*55-64*	*65+*
New Orleans, U.S.A. (all groups)	5.1	4.3	6.7	7.2
Cali, Colombia	3.3	3.3	3.6	4.0

TABLE 11–12 Prevalence Rate (%) of Multiple Polyps by Age, Sex, and Location

	Age		
	15–44	*45–64*	*65+*
New Orleans, U.S.A.			
White males	–	23.6	21.9
White females	–	11.4	13.3
Black males	3.0	13.1	33.0
Black females	–	14.5	15.4
Cali, Colombia			
Males	0.6	3.9	11.9
Females	–	2.1	3.4

New Orleans and Cali, and shows clearly that the size of polyps increases with age and is considerably greater in patients living in New Orleans than in those of Cali. No sex- or race-related differences are demonstrated in either city. This greater frequency and greater size of adenomatous polyps in New Orleans compared with Cali parallels the increase of colon cancer rates with age and the greater frequency of colon cancer in New Orleans as compared with Cali. It is well-known from other studies that larger polyps run a greater risk of developing atypias and malignant transformations, and that the risk of cancer increases with the number of adenomatous polyps (Arminski and McLean, 1964; Morson, 1974).

An indication of the frequency of multiple polyps for individuals living in Cali and New Orleans is given in Table 11–12 in the form of prevalence rates of multiple polyps, representing the number of persons bearing two or more polyps divided by the number of colons examined. The rate of multiple tumors is several times greater in New Orleans than it is in Cali. It is also somewhat higher in males in all groups, possibly indicating an earlier response to tumorigenic influences in males.

Sato and co-workers (1976) in Japan have shown that the prevalence of multiple polyps was higher in Akita prefecture than in Miyagi, where colon cancer is less frequent than in Akita (13.7 per cent versus 7.5 per cent). Polyps on the average were larger in individuals from Akita than in those from Miyagi; 27 per cent of adenomatous polyps were greater than 4.9 mm in diameter in Akita versus 16 per cent in Miyagi.

We have, therefore, an increased frequency of multiple tumors and an increase in size in polyps in individuals living in New Orleans as compared with those living in Cali, and in Akita as compared with Miyagi. This difference is independent from the differences in the number of persons affected by polyps in each community (prevalence rate). A higher proportion of individuals is affected by polyps in populations with higher cancer risks. Furthermore, those affected seem to have a greater dose of the tumorigenic stimulus, as measured by the increase in number of polyps and the increase in size of polyps.

Sato and co-workers also evaluated the degree of histologic (architectural) and cytologic atypia in adenomatous polyps. They found that 23 per cent of polyps studied in Akita had moderate or severe atypia, whereas only 12.7 per cent of those from Miyagi showed these changes. Our model (Haenszel and Correa, 1971) postulates that the distal colon receives a greater dose of carcinogen than the proximal colon. This is supported by the findings of Japanese (Sato et al., 1976) and Swedish (Prager et al., 1974) investigators who have reported that polyps of the distal (sigmoid) colon have more advanced atypical and dysplastic changes than those of the proximal (cecum) colon.

BIOLOGIC SOUNDNESS

There are many studies of the biologic aspects of adenomatous polyps and colon cancer bearing on the coherence of the polyp-cancer sequence concept, reviewed in other sections of this monograph. Observations in patients with adenomatous polyps have documented the progression from benign to atypical to malignant epithelial changes (Morson, 1974). Experimental studies have shown that several carcinogens produce adenomatous polyps and carcinomas morphologically identical with those observed in humans (Spjut and Spratt, 1965).

Causality

From the foregoing discussion it is hard to escape the conclusion that adenomatous polyps and colon adenocarcinoma are causally associated. If we are dealing with a directly causal association, we should expect adenomatous polyps to be a prerequisite to the appearance of carcinomas. In the cases in which carcinomas arise in previously existing adenomatous polyps, which seem to be the majority (Morson, 1974), we will have to admit a directly causal association. In the hypothetical cases of carcinoma originating in the intestinal mucosa not previously replaced by an adenomatous polyp (Spratt and Ackerman, 1962), it would seem that both lesions are related to a third cause, and therefore the association would be indirectly causal. The distinction between direct and indirect causality has relevance as it relates to the management of polyps. A report of a 15-year follow-up of patients with adenomatous polyps removed after sigmoidoscopy indicates that the risk of colon cancer in these patients is twice the expected frequency. The cancers found were in segments of the bowel that were too high for diagnosis and treatment by proctosigmoidoscopy (Prager et al., 1974). It seems, therefore, that a number of cancers were prevented by the resection of these polyps. The ideal of prevention, however, should include the prevention of adenomas, and if that could be accomplished the distinction between direct and indirect causality would be irrelevant.

The epidemiologic evidence accumulated indicates that the same etiologic factors are associated with adenomatous polyps and colon cancer. The removal of those factors from a community, therefore, should result in drastic reductions in the frequency of both benign and malignant expressions of the neoplastic process. Since adenomatous polyps are a good indicator of colon cancer risk, it should be expected that individuals with polyps are exposed to the same factors that lead ultimately to cancer. They should provide fruitful clues to epidemiologists and should be useful to test hypotheses derived from cancer patients, such as those related to the amount of bulk, fat, and meat in the diet as well as those related to the fecal flora and fecal steroid conversion rates. The problem with these types of studies is to find adequate controls, which should be free of polyps. Unfortunately there is no practical method available today to rule out the presence of very small adenomatous polyps in living subjects, except perhaps the somewhat involved procedure of fiberoptic colonoscopy.

Ekelund, utilizing radiologic methods, found that 7 per cent of 115 subjects who were previously free of polyps developed them after eight or more years of observation. None of them developed carcinoma. An equal number of patients with polyps were followed for approximately the same time; of these, 21 per cent developed new polyps and 2.7 per cent developed carcinomas. These differences are statistically significant (Brahme et al., 1974). Studies of fecal flora have so far revealed no differences between the flora of polyp-free patients and polyp-bearers (Finegold et al., 1975; Moore and Holdeman, 1975), but the complexity of fecal bacteriology should not be overlooked. It is still premature to rule out differences in the taxonomy and functions of the fecal bacteria between polyp-bearers and polyp-free individuals.

The appearance of new adenomatous polyps in a patient probably reflects the action of "initiating" factors, whereas the increase in size of polyps and the atypia probably reflects "promoting" factors. It is not known if the initiators and the promoters are the same or different factors. Experimental studies suggest that some carcinogens are initiators and promoters at the same time. The similarity of the epidemiology of colon cancer and adenomatous polyps points in the direction of similarities between initiators and promoters.

CONCLUSIONS

There is a very close parallel in the epidemiology of colon cancer and adenomatous polyps. Both conditions are strongly related to geography, anatomic localization, socioeconomic class, migration experience, and time trends. The strength of the association favors the notion of a direct, positive correlation between multiple tumors, size and atypia of polyps, and cancer risks, equivalent to "dose-effect." The epidemiologic findings are coherent with other biologic facts derived from clinical, morphologic, and experimental studies. Adenomatous polyps are a good epidemiologic indicator of colon cancer risk, and their presence should be helpful in advancing from studies of the epidemiology of colon cancer to the epidemiology of precursor lesions.

No epidemiologic support for a precancerous role of juvenile polyps has been found. The epidemiology of hyperplastic polyps suggests environmental factors independent of those associated with colon cancer.

References

Andren, L., and Frieberg, S.: Frequency of polyps of the rectum and colon, according to age, and relation to cancer. Acta Radiol. *46*:631, 1956.

Arminski, T. C., and McLean, D. W.: Incidence and distribution of adenomatous polyps of the colon and rectum based on 1000 autopsy examinations. Dis. Colon Rectum *7*:249, 161, 1964.

Arthur, J. F.: Structure and significance of metaplastic nodules in the rectal mucosa. J. Clin. Pathol. *21*:735, 1968.

Axtell, L. M., and Chiazze, L., Jr.: Changing relative frequency of cancers of the colon and rectum in the United States. Cancer *19*:750, 1966.

Berg, J. W., and Haenszel, W.: Epidemiology of cancer of the lower colon and rectum. In preparation for publication.

Berg, J. W., and Howell, M. A.: The geographic pathology of large bowel cancer. Cancer *134*(Suppl.):807, 1974.

Blatt, L. J.: Polyps of the colon and rectum: Incidence and distribution. Dis. Colon Rectum *4*:277, 1961.

Bone, E., Drasar, B. S., and Hill, M. J.: Gut bacteria and their metabolic activities in familial polyposis. Lancet *1*:1117, 1975.

Brahme, F., Ekelund, G. R., Norden, J. G., and Wenckest, A.: Metachronous colorectal polyps. A comparison between the development of colorectal polyps and carcinomas in persons with and without polyps in their history. Dis. Colon Rectum *17*:166, 1974.

Bremner, C. G., and Ackerman, L. V.: Polyps and carcinoma of the large bowel in the South African Bantu. Cancer *26*:991, 1970.

Burkitt, D. P.: Epidemiology of cancer of the colon and rectum. Cancer *28*:3, 1971.

Cady, B., Persson, A. V., Monson, D. O., and Maunz, D.: Changing patterns of colorectal carcinoma. Cancer *33*:423, 1974.

Cole, J. W.: 2, 3 Dimethyl-4-aminobiphenyl: absence of carcinogenicity in germ-free rats. Quoted by Wynder, E. L., Kajitani, T., Ishikawa, S., Dodo, H., and Takano, A.: Environmental factors in cancer of the colon and rectum. Cancer *23*:1210, 1969.

Correa, P.: Comments on the epidemiology of large bowel cancer. Cancer Res. *35*:3395, 1975.

Correa, P., Duque, E., Cuello, C., and Haenszel, W.: Polyps of the colon and rectum in Cali, Colombia. Int. J. Cancer *9*:86, 1972.

Cutler, S. J., and Devesa, S. S.: Trends in cancer incidence and mortality in the U.S.A. *In* Host-environment interactions in the etiology of cancer in man. IARC Scientific Publication, No. 7, Lyon, 1973, pp:15–34.

Cutler, S. J., and Young, J. L.: Third National Cancer Survey. Incidence data. Natl. Cancer Inst. Monograph 41, 1975.

Doll, R., Muir, C. S., and Waterhouse, J. A. H. (eds.): Cancer Incidence in Five Continents, Vol. 2. UICC, Geneva, 1970.

Dorn, H. F., and Cutler, S. J.: Morbidity from cancer in the U.S. U.S. Public Health Service Monograph No. 56, Washington, D.C., 1959.
Ekelund, G., and Lindstrom, C.: Histopathologic analysis of benign polyps in patients with carcinoma of the colon and rectum. Gut *15*:654, 1974.
Finegold, S. M., Flora, D. J., Atterby, H. A., and Sutter, V. L.: Fecal bacteriology of colonic polyp patients and control patients. Cancer Res. *35*:3407, 1975.
Gennaro, A. R., Villanueva, R., Sokonthaman, Y., Vathanophos, V., and Rosemond, G. P.: Chemical carcinogenesis in transposed intestinal segments. Cancer Res. *33*:536, 1973.
Haenszel, W.: Cancer mortality among the foreign born in the United States. J. Natl. Cancer Inst. *26*:37, 1961.
Haenszel, W., and Berg, J. W.: Large bowel cancer in Hawaii Japanese. J. Natl. Cancer Inst., *51*:1765, 1973.
Haenszel, W., and Correa, P.: Cancer of the colon and rectum and adenomatous polyps. A review of epidemiologic findings. Cancer *28*:14, 1971.
Haenszel, W., and Correa, P.: Cancer of the large intestine: epidemiologic findings. Dis. Colon Rectum *16*:371, 1973.
Haenszel, W., Correa, P., and Cuello, C.: Social class differences in large bowel cancer in Cali, Colombia. J. Natl. Cancer Inst. *54*:1031, 1975.
Haenszel, W., and Kurihara, M.: Studies of Japanese migrants. I. Mortality from cancer and other diseases among Japanese in the United States. J. Natl. Cancer Inst. *40*:43, 1968.
Helwig, E. B.: Adenomas of large intestine in children. Am. J. Dis. Child *72*:289, 1946.
Helwig, E. B.: The evolution of adenomas of the large intestine and their relationship to carcinoma. Surg. Gynecol. Obstet. *84*:36, 1947.
Hill, M. J.: Steroid nuclear dehydrogenation and colon cancer. Am. J. Clin. Nutr. *27*:1475, 1974a.
Hill, M. J.: Colon cancer. A disease of fibre depletion or of dietary excess? Digestion *11*: 289, 1974b.
Hill, M. J., Crowther, J. S., Drasar, B. S., Hawksworth, G., Aries, V., and Williams, R. E. O.: Bacteria and the etiology of cancer of large bowel. Lancet *1*:95, 1971.
Lane, N., Kaplan, H., and Pascal, R.: Minute adenomatous and hyperplastic polyps of the colon: divergent patterns of epithelial growth with specific associated mesenchymal changes. Gastroenterology *60*:537, 1971.
Laqueur, G. L.: Contribution of Intestinal Macroflora and Microflora to Carcinogenesis. *In* Burdette, W. J. (ed.): Carcinoma of the Colon and Antecedent Epithelium. Charles C Thomas, Springfield, Ill., 1970.
Marigo, C.: Personal communication. São Paulo, Brazil.
Moore, W. E. C., and Holdeman, C. V.: Discussion of current bacteriological investigations of the relationship between intestinal flora, diet and colon cancer. Cancer Res. *35*:3418, 1975.
Morson, B. C.: Some peculiarities in the histology of intestinal polyps. Dis. Colon Rectum *5*:337, 1962.
Morson, B. C.: The polyp-cancer sequence in the large bowel. Proc. R. Soc. Med. *67*:451, 1974.
Moya de Madrigal, L.: Cancer of the alimentary tract in Costa Rica. Pan American Health Organization Bulletin *8*:150, 1974.
Prager, E. D., Swinton, N. W., Young, J., Veidenheimer, M. C., and Corman, M. L.: Follow-up study of patients with benign mucosal polyps discovered by proctosigmoidoscopy. Dis. Colon Rectum *17*:322, 1974.
Puffer, R., and Griffith, G. W.: Patterns of urban mortality. Pan American Health Organization. Scientific Publication No. 151, Washington, D.C., 1967.
Restrepo, C.: Personal communication, Medellín, Colombia.
Rose, G., Blackburn, H., Keys, A., Taylor, H. L., Kannel, W. B., Paul, O., Reid, D. D., and Stamler, J.: Colon cancer and blood cholesterol. Lancet *1*:181, 1974.
Roth, S. I., and Helwig, E. B.: Juvenile polyps of the colon and rectum. Cancer *16*:468, 1963.
Sato, E., Ouchi, A., Sasano, N., and Ishidate, T.: Polyps and diverticulosis of large bowel in autopsy population of Akita prefecture: high risk to colrectal cancer in Japan, compared with Miyagi. Cancer, *37*:1316, 1976.
Segura, J. J.: Personal communication, San José, Costa Rica.
Spjut, H. J., and Spratt, J. S., Jr.: Endemic and morphologic similarities existing be-

tween spontaneous colonic neoplasms in man and 3:2′ dimethyl-4-aminobiphenyl induced colonic neoplasms in rats. Ann. Surg. *161*:309, 1965.

Spratt, J. S., and Ackerman, L. V.: Small primary adenocarcinomas of the colon and rectum. J.A.M.A. *179*:337, 1962.

Staszewski, J., and Haenszel, W.: Cancer mortality among the Polish born in the United States. J. Natl. Cancer Inst. *35*:291, 1965.

Stemmermann, G. N.: Cancer of the colon and rectum discovered at autopsy in Hawaiian Japanese. Cancer *19*:1567, 1966.

Stemmermann, G. N., and Yatani, R.: Diverticulosis and polyps of the large intestine. Cancer *31*:1260, 1973.

Ward, J. M., Yamamoto, R. J., and Brown, C.: Pathology of intestinal neoplasms and other lesions in rats exposed to azoxymethane. J. Natl. Cancer Inst. *51*:1029, 1973.

Wilkins, T. D.: Personal communication.

Williams, A. O., Chung, E. B., Aghata, A., and Jackson, M. A.: Intestinal polyps in American negroes and Nigerian Africans. Br. J. Cancer *31*:485, 1975.

Wynder, E. L.: The epidemiology of large bowel cancer. Cancer Res. *35*:3388, 1975.

Chapter Twelve

Etiology of the Adenoma-Carcinoma Sequence

Michael Hill

INTRODUCTION

The evidence given in previous chapters suggests that most carcinomas of the large bowel arise in adenomas. In any investigation of the etiology of large bowel cancer, therefore, it would seem sensible to study the cause of the principal predisposing conditions. In practice this is very difficult, and most of our knowledge of the incidence of adenomas in various populations is deduced by analogy from our knowledge of the incidence of carcinoma in those populations.

In this chapter the current position is outlined and a postulated etiology of adenomas is presented. This inevitably points the way to further studies, and some of these, too, will be discussed. The one fact that overwhelms any serious discussion of this subject is the dearth of hard data, and thus a good deal of speculation is inevitable.

THE EPIDEMIOLOGY OF ADENOMAS

The epidemiology of adenomas has been discussed in Chapter 11. In summary the indications are that both the proportion of persons carrying adenomas and the number of adenomas per carrier are lower in Africa, Asia, and South America than in North America and Northwest Europe. Good data on incidence rates are available from only a few countries but, until it is proved otherwise, we can deduce a more generalized statement from the geographic distribution of large bowel cancer.

The Geographic Distribution of Adenomas

It is known that the incidence of adenomas in Japanese living in Japan (Sato, 1974) is lower than that in Japanese born in Hawaii (Stemmermann and Yatani, 1976). The incidence of adenomas in black Africans is very low indeed (Bremner and Ackerman, 1970; Williams et al., 1975), whereas that in black Americans is as high as in white Americans. Thus the incidence rates in populations generally do not differ because of a difference in genetic constitution, but because of some environmental factor.

It is clear from the few comparable studies carried out that although, in general, carriage of intestinal adenomas parallels the incidence of intestinal cancer, this relationship is by no means a simple one. In three countries with low incidences of large bowel cancer, the incidence of adenomas varies from almost zero (black South Africans) to 10 per cent in Japan and in Cali, Colombia. Thus, the presence of adenomas does not necessarily imply a proportionate risk of large bowel cancer. This may be due to differences in size of adenomas.

Size of Adenomas in Various Populations

In this field too there have been very few studies, but these indicate that the adenomas in Japan and Colombia are small, with very few larger than 1 cm in diameter. In their study of Japanese adenomas, Muto et al. (1977) found the same relation between adenoma size and malignant potential as did Morson (1974) in London and Berge et al. (1973) in Sweden (Table 12–1). However, only 5 per cent of the Japanese adenomas were greater than 1 cm in diameter (Table 12–2), and only 2 per cent of adenomas reported in Cali, Colombia, were greater than this size (Correa et al., 1972); the low incidence of large bowel cancer in these two countries, therefore, could be directly related to the small numbers of large adenomas rather than to the total number of all adenomas in these studies.

In Sweden, in contrast, the size distribution of adenomas was similar to that in the United States and Britain (Berge et al., 1973); the carriage

TABLE 12–1 The Relation Between Size and Malignant Potential of Adenomas in Three Countries

Size of Adenoma	% With Malignancy *Japan*	*England*	*Sweden*
< 1 cm	1.0	1.3	3.6
1–2 cm	9.8	9.5	59.0 (1–2 cm and > 2 cm combined)
> 2 cm	41.7	46.0	

TABLE 12–2 The Proportion of Adenomas Greater than 1 cm in Diameter in Five Populations

Population	% of Adenomas Greater than 1 cm in Diameter	Reference
England	39	Morson, 1974
Sweden	27	Berge et al., 1973
Colombia	2	Correa et al., 1972
U.S.A.	15	Arminski and McLean, 1964
Japan	5	Sato, 1974

rate of all adenomas is similar to that in Britain so that, again, the risk of large bowel cancer can be related to the incidence of large adenomas. If this is so, we can tentatively extrapolate the data on the geographic distribution of large bowel cancer to imply the same geographic distribution of *large* adenomas.

Subsite Distribution of Adenomas

Studies based on autopsy data or on colonoscopy show a fairly even distribution of adenomas in the large bowel (Table 12–3). For example, Ekelund (1963) found that in Malmö, out of 498 large bowel adenomas, 24 per cent were in the cecum and ascending colon, 30 per cent in the transverse and descending colon, 30 per cent in the sigmoid colon, and 16 per cent in the rectum; similar results have been obtained in Colombia and in the United States (Table 12–3), and in a further three studies of autopsy material (Feyrter, 1931; Lawrence, 1936; Blatt, 1961). There is a very different distribution of carcinomas; for example, in the Malmö study 65 per cent of the carcinomas were located in the sigmoid colon and rectum compared with only 46 per cent of the polyps; similar differences have been documented in Colombia and the United States (Correa et al., 1972).

TABLE 12–3 Subsite Distribution of Adenomas Based on Autopsy Data from Three Populations

Subsite	Sweden[1]	Colombia[2]	U.S.A.[3]
Cecum and ascending colon	24	18	24
Transverse and descending colon	30	41	35
Sigmoid colon	30	20	22
Rectum	16	21	19

[1]*From* Ekelund, G., 1963.
[2]*From* Correa, P., et al., 1972.
[3]*From* Arminski, T. C., and McLean, D. W., 1964.

There are few published data on the subsite distribution of large adenomas, but we can deduce from the data on the relation between the malignant potential and the size of adenomas that the distribution of large adenomas will be similar to that of the carcinomas. Thus, the adenomas on the right side will be predominantly small, whereas those on the left will include most of the large adenomas present; this was found by Sato (1974) to be true for Japanese adenomas.

Genetic Aspects of Adenoma Carriage

Adenomatosis (also known as familial polyposis coli) is undoubtedly a genetically determined disease, being due to a non-sex-linked dominant gene transmitted on normal mendelian lines. By analogy Veale (1965), a geneticist, put forward the suggestion that in fact all adenomas have a genetic etiology. He proposed that, if the normal gene is designated "+", and the gene for small numbers of adenomas is "p", then persons with the combination "++" will not carry adenomas; similarly those who are "p+" will also appear normal and carry no adenomas, but those who are "pp" will develop adenomas.

To date this hypothesis has not been tested, and so there is no direct evidence either to support or to refute it. However, there is some indirect evidence since Lovett (1974) has shown that siblings of large bowel cancer patients have an incidence of large bowel cancer many times that expected. The study was based on a moderate number of patients, but needs to be repeated elsewhere. However, if large bowel cancer is familial, it could be inferred that adenomas also have a familial etiology.

POSTULATED ETIOLOGY OF ADENOMAS

If we accept that the ability to produce adenomas of the large bowel is genetically determined, we need to know the distribution of the gene in the population. If we assume that in the West all adenoma-prone persons (i.e., those who are "pp" on Veale's notation) actually develop adenomas, then the gene is extremely widespread. It is also as common in Japanese and Negroes as in Caucasians, since the black, white, and Japanese populations of the United States have similar incidences of adenomas. Data in the literature would indicate that we have still to see the full expression of the adenoma-prone gene, since the incidence of adenomas appears still to be increasing in the United States (Correa et al., 1972). However, this may be due to changes in diagnostic technique, the use of the hand lens inevitably increasing the number of small adenomas detected. In the study by Stemmermann and Yatani (1976), more than 60 per cent of Japanese born in Hawaii had adenomas, and would therefore be "pp"; in order to maintain this high proportion virtually all of the remainder would have to be "p+", and "++" persons would need to be very rare (5 per cent or less of the population).

In order to explain the difference in incidence of adenomas between the Japanese living in Japan and those living in Hawaii, there must be a further factor of an environmental nature that determines whether an adenoma-prone person actually develops adenomas. This environmental factor, "E_1", must be abundant in the West and presumably ensures that virtually all "pp" persons develop adenomas if they have a western way of life; it must be virtually absent from the environment of the African Bantu (since adenomas are so rare among them), and must be at intermediate levels in the Japanese and Colombian environment.

This environmental factor would explain the variation in incidence rates of adenomas per se, but would not explain why so few of the Japanese or Colombian adenomas grow to a size greater than 1 cm in diameter compared with those in British, Swedish, or American persons. For this we must postulate a further factor; since a high proportion of adenomas grow to a large size in Japanese living in Hawaii, but not in those living in Japan, there must be a second environmental factor, "E_2".

We now have a postulated scheme for the etiology of intestinal adenomas and their further growth (Fig. 12–1). Since the same proportion of large adenomas become malignant in Japanese in Japan as in western populations, we do not necessarily need a further factor to explain the progression to malignancy; if such a factor exists, it must be ubiquitous throughout the world. For the sake of completeness a factor has been postulated which is able to produce malignancy in adenomatous tissue; obviously, the larger the amount of adenomatous tissue, the greater the risk of malignancy. If carcinoma de novo arises it is due to the effect of "C" on normal colorectal mucosal tissue. The evident rarity of such events indicates that the normal tissue is much less sensitive to "C" than is adenomatous tissue. This factor would presumably be the "carcinogen," and so has been referred to as factor "C"; since its distribution is so even, it need not be considered further as a determinant in the incidence of adenoma or carcinoma.

How does this postulate fit the available data? In Table 12–4 the data for Britain, America, Colombia, Sweden, Japan, South Africa, and Nigeria are fitted to the postulate. Since the adenoma-prone genetic factor is widespread in black Americans, it is presumably as common in their black African forebears; thus, factor "E_1" must be absent from the environment of black Africans, and, in the absence of the precursor adenomas, nothing can be deduced about the amount of environmental factor "E_2".

Since Japanese in the United States have a high incidence of adenomas, they must have the usual high level of the genetic factor "pp". Since adenomas are produced in 10 per cent of Japanese living in Japan,

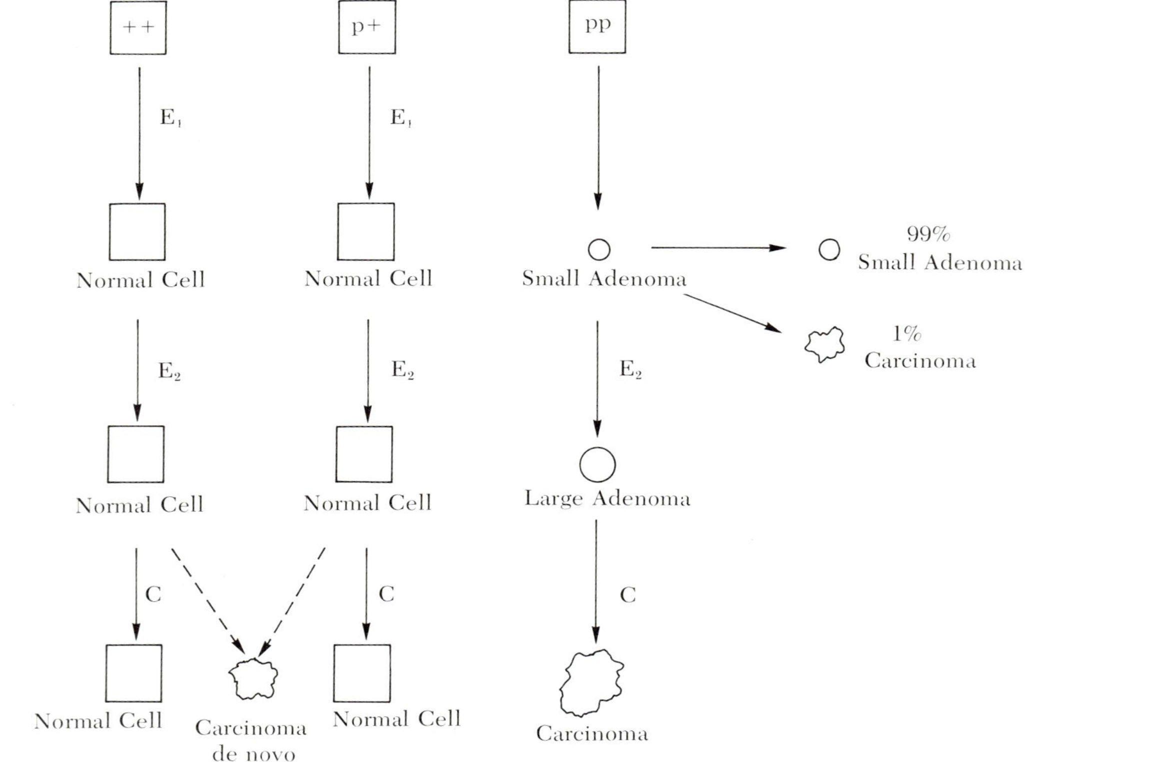

Figure 12–1 Postulated mechanism for the progression of normal tissue to adenoma to carcinoma pp is the recessive gene conferring "adenoma-prone" status. E_1 is the environmental factor that causes the formation of adenomas in adenoma-prone persons. E_2 is the environmental factor that causes adenomas to grow. C is the carcinogen responsible for the progression of adenoma to carcinoma, and possibly for the de novo production of carcinoma in normal cells.

TABLE 12–4 The Prevalence in Various Countries of the Various Factors Postulated in the Causation of Large Bowel Cancer, Deduced from Data on the Incidence of Adenomas and of Large Bowel Cancer

	Proportion pp	Factor E_1	Factor E_2	Factor C
Cali	+++	+	−	+
Nigeria	+++	−	?	+
Johannesburg, black	+++	−	?	+
U.S., black	+++	+++	+++	+
Japan	+++	+	−	+
Japanese in U.S.	+++	+++	+++	+
Sweden	+++	+++	+++	+
Britain	+++	+++	+++	+
U.S., white	+++	+++	+++	+

there must be a moderate amount of factor "E_1" in the Japanese environment; since the adenomas are nearly all small we can deduce that factor "E_2" must be virtually absent. The situation in Cali is similar; the level of "E_1" must be similar to that in Japan, and "E_2" must be virtually absent.

We have a relative abundance of data on the incidence of large bowel cancer. Populations with a high incidence must have high levels of both "E_1" and "E_2", as well as the normal high proportion of adenoma-prone persons. A low incidence, however, could be due to low levels of either "E_1" or "E_2", or both. It could also be due to a low proportion of adenoma-prone persons in the population. Thus a population such as Finland, which has a western way of life, and in particular a western-style high fat and high meat diet, might be expected to have a "western" level of "E_2". The low incidence of large bowel cancer therefore, on this postulate, would be due to a very low incidence of adenomas; however, we would expect a high proportion of these to be large because of the high level of "E_2". The very low incidence of adenomas could be due to a low proportion of the population being adenoma-prone (possible in a population away from the genetic mainstream), or to a low level of "E_1". The proportion of adenomas progressing to malignancy would be expected to be high.

The Nature of E_1, E_2, and C

If the postulated mechanism for the causation of adenomas and their progression to carcinoma is correct, then from our knowledge of adenomas we should be able to deduce something of the nature of the causative agents.

Adenomas are fairly evenly distributed along the large intestine. If the effect of the genetic factor is to make the whole of the large intestine equally adenoma-prone, the environmental factor "E_1" must also be fairly evenly distributed. DeCosse et al. (1975) have reported that regression of adenomas may be achieved by treatment with luminal ascorbic acid. These studies are very preliminary, but if the results are confirmed they imply that "E_1" is also luminal *and* that it is sensitive to oxidation by ascorbate. It has been suggested that rectal adenomas in patients with adenomatosis also regress following colectomy; if this is true it would also support the luminal nature of "E_1". Interestingly, both of these latter studies indicate that adenomas not only are caused by "E_1", but need a constant supply of it to maintain their integrity, and that removal of it from the environment would cause regression of the adenomas and, therefore, a reduction in the incidence of large bowel cancer.

Since adenomas are as common in the right colon as in the left, "E_1" is not a product of gut bacterial metabolism (unless it is the product of a very rapid reaction in the cecum, such as the hydrolysis of a glycoside). Conversely, since polyps are as common in the left as in the right colon, "E_1" is not sensitive to microbial degradation. In summary, from the limited data available on the incidence of adenomas in various parts of the world, "E_1" is a luminal factor ingested only in a preformed state or enterohepatically circulated following airborne ingestion; it is sensitive to ascorbic acid but is not metabolized by the gut flora; it must be continuously available for the adenoma to develop and to be maintained.

"E_2" is almost certainly the factor investigated in studies of the etiology of large bowel cancer. Large adenomas progress to carcinoma in the same proportion in Japan as in Britain and Sweden, indicating that the malignant potential of large adenomas is constant in high and low large bowel cancer incidence areas; thus epidemiologic deductions on the basis of large bowel cancer incidence data will also apply to large adenomas. If this is true, "E_2" is at a higher concentration in the left colon than in the right colon; is at a higher concentration in the large bowel of social class I than in that of social class IV and V persons; is related to the intake of dietary fat and meat; and is possibly the same bacterial metabolite of the bile acids incriminated in the etiology of large bowel cancer (Hill et al., 1975; Hill, 1975). Indeed, the combination of high fecal bile acid concentration and the presence of certain clostridia should characterize a high proportion of persons with large adenomas, as it does those with large bowel cancer (Hill et al., 1975). This is currently being investigated.

Since the proportion of large adenomas progressing to carcinoma is the same in Japan as in Britain and Sweden, factor "C" must be fairly uniformly distributed, and plays no role in determining the rate of progression from adenoma to carcinoma. The postulate is that, although factor "C" is potentially able to induce malignancy in any cell, the large adenoma is extremely sensitive to factor "C" (since at least one-half of them become malignant), the small adenoma is much less sensitive (since only about 1 per cent of small adenomas become malignant), and normal tissue is very insensitive (since carcinoma de novo has still to be proved to the satisfaction of most pathologists). It is likely that all adenomatous tissue is equally sensitive to "C", and that the difference in malignant potential between adenomas of different size is due to the difference in the mass of adenomatous tissue. Factor "C" may not be a single entity; a wide range of carcinogens is ingested from various sources (diet, polluted air, etc.), but only those reaching the colon in an active form would be relevant to this discussion.

CONCLUSIONS

If this postulate is correct, it has certain implications. The first is that the development of adenomas is dependent on two factors, one genetic and one environmental. In general, the genetic factor must be fairly evenly distributed geographically, but there may be populations in which the proportion of adenoma-prone persons is small. If such a population has a western life-style, the incidence of adenomas would still be low, although all adenoma-prone persons would develop them; however, the proportion of adenomas progressing to become large adenomas, and then to carcinomas, would be as high as in other western countries. This gives a cancer incidence below that expected from the life-style, but above that expected from a comparison of the incidence of all colorectal adenomas with that in Japan and in Britain. Finland might be such a country, and a study of colorectal adenomas in Finland would be of great interest.

On this postulate no population with a non-western life-style would be expected to have a high incidence of large adenomas (and therefore of large bowel cancer); to date no such population is known, but if one with a low meat/low fat diet was found to have a high incidence of the disease, this would call for gross revision, or rejection, of the postulate.

Finally, this postulated etiology can only be judged when we have much more data on the incidence of adenomas, their size distribution, and their malignant potential in a large number of populations with high and low incidences of large bowel cancer.

It is ironic that, although a full understanding of the etiology of colorectal adenomas would be invaluable in the study of the causation of cancer, we have far more data on the latter than the former, and have to deduce so much about adenomas from our knowledge of carcinomas.

References

Arminski, T. C., and McLean, D. W.: Incidence and distribution of adenomatous polyps of the colon and rectum based on 1,000 autopsy examinations. Dis. Colon Rectum 7:249, 1964.

Berge, T., Ekelund, G., Mellner, C., Pihl, B., and Wenckert, A.: Carcinoma of the colon and rectum in a defined population. Acta Chir. Scand (Suppl. 438), 1973.

Blatt, L. J.: Polyps of the colon and rectum. Incidence and distribution. Dis. Colon Rectum *4*:277, 1961.

Bremner, C. G., and Ackerman, L. V.: Polyps and carcinoma of the large bowel in the South African Bantu. Cancer *26*:991, 1970.

Correa, P., Duque, E., Cuello, C., and Haenszel, W.: Polyps of the colon and rectum in Cali, Colombia. Br. J. Cancer *9*:86, 1972.

DeCosse, J. J., Adams, M. B., Kuzma, J. F., Logerfo, P., and Condon, R. E.: The effect of ascorbic acid on rectal polyps of patients with familial polyposis. Surgery *78*:608, 1975.

Ekelund, G.: On cancer and polyps of colon and rectum. Acta Pathol. Microbiol. Scand. *59*:165, 1963.

Feyrter, F.: Zur Geschwulstlehre (nach Untersuchungen am menschlichen Darm). Beitr. Pathol. Anat. *77*:1852, 1931.

Hill, M. J.: The etiology of colon cancer. Crit. Rev. Toxicol. *4*:31, 1975.

Hill, M. J., Drasar, B. S., Williams, R. E. O., Meade, T. W., Cox, A. G., Simpson, J. E. P., and Morson, B. C.: Faecal bile acids and clostridia in patients with cancer of the large bowel. Lancet *1*:535, 1975.

Lawrence, J. C.: Gastrointestinal polyps. Statistical study of malignancy incidence. Am. J. Surg. *31*:499, 1936.

Lovett, E.: Familial factors in the etiology of carcinoma of the bowel. Proc. R. Soc. Med. *67*:751, 1974.

Morson, B.: The polyp cancer sequence in the large bowel. Proc. R. Soc. Med. *67*:451, 1974.

Muto, T., Ishikawa, K., Kino, I., Nakamura, K., Sugano, H., Morson, B. C., and Bussey, H. J. R.: Comparative histological study of large bowel adenomas in Japan and England with special reference to malignant potential. Dis. Colon Rectum, *20*:11, 1977.

Sato, E.: Adenomatous polyps of large intestine in autopsy and surgical material. Gann *65*:295, 1974.

Stemmermann, G. N., and Yatani, R.: Diverticulosis and polyps of the large intestine. Cancer *31*:1260, 1976.

Veale, A. M. O.: Intestinal Polyposis. Eugenics Laboratory Memoirs, Series 40, Cambridge University Press, London, 1965.

Williams, A. O., Chung, E. B., Agbata, A., and Jackson, M.: Intestinal polyps in American Negroes and Nigerian Africans. Br. J. Cancer *31*:485, 1975.

INDEX

Page numbers in *italic type* refer to illustrations.